Baillière's

CLINICAL
OBSTETRICS
AND
GYNAECOLOGY

INTERNATIONAL PRACTICE AND RESEARCH

Baillière's

CLINICAL OBSTETRICS AND GYNAECOLOGY

INTERNATIONAL PRACTICE AND RESEARCH

Volume 5/Number 4
December 1991

Hormone Replacement and its Impact on Osteoporosis

C. CHRISTIANSEN MD
Guest Editor

Baillière Tindall
London Philadelphia Sydney Tokyo Toronto

This book is printed on acid-free paper.

Baillière Tindall 24–28 Oval Road,
W.B. Saunders London NW1 7DX

The Curtis Center, Independence Square West,
Philadelphia, PA 19106–3399, USA

55 Horner Avenue
Toronto, Ontario M8Z 4X6, Canada

Harcourt Brace Jovanovich Group (Australia) Pty Ltd,
30–52 Smidmore Street, Marrickville, NSW 2204, Australia

Harcourt Brace Jovanovich Japan, Inc,
Ichibancho Central Building,
22-1 Ichibancho, Chiyoda-ku, Tokyo 102, Japan

ISSN 0950–3552

ISBN 0–7020–1548–2 (single copy)

Baillière's Clinical Obstetrics and Gynaecology is published four times each year by
Baillière Tindall. Annual subscription prices are:

TERRITORY	ANNUAL SUBSCRIPTION	SINGLE ISSUE
1. UK	£55.00 post free	£27.50 post free
2. Europe	£61.00 post free	£27.50 post free
3. All other countries	Consult your local Harcourt Brace Jovanovich office for dollar price	

The editor of this publication is Margaret Macdonald, Baillière Tindall,
24–28 Oval Road, London NW1 7DX.

Baillière's Clinical Obstetrics and Gynaecology was published from 1983 to 1986 as
Clinics in Obstetrics and Gynaecology.

Typeset by Phoenix Photosetting, Chatham.
Printed and bound in Great Britain by Mackays of Chatham PLC, Chatham, Kent.

Contributors to this issue

MICHAEL R. ADAMS DVM, Associate Professor of Comparative Medicine, Bowman Gray School of Medicine of Wake Forest University, Winston-Salem, NC 27103, USA.

TRUDY L. BUSH PhD, MHS, Department of Epidemiology, The Johns Hopkins University/SHPH, 615 N. Wolfe Street, Room 6029, Baltimore, MD 21205, USA.

CHARLES H. CHESNUT III MD, Professor of Medicine, Radiology and Nutritional Sciences; Adjunct Professor, Orthopaedics; Director, Osteoporosis Research Center, University of Washington Medical Center, Seattle, Washington 98195, USA.

CLAUS CHRISTIANSEN MD, Department of Clinical Chemistry, Glostrup Hospital, University of Copenhagen, DK-2600 Glostrup, Denmark.

THOMAS B. CLARKSON DVM, Professor and Chairman of Comparative Medicine; Director, Arteriosclerosis Research Center and Comparative Medicine Research Center, Bowman Gray School of Medicine of Wake Forest University, 300 South Hawthorne Road, Winston-Salem, NC 27103, USA.

STEVEN R. CUMMINGS MD, Associate Professor of Medicine and Epidemiology, Divisions of General Internal Medicine and Clinical Epidemiology, University of California, San Francisco, California, USA.

PIERRE D. DELMAS MD, PhD, Professor of Medicine and Rheumatology, University Claude Bernard of Lyon, Department of Rheumatology and Bone Disease and INSERM Unit 234, Ed. Herroit Hospital, 69437 Lyon Cedex 03, France.

CHRISTIAN HASSAGER MD, PhD, Department of Clinical Chemistry, Glostrup Hospital, University of Copenhagen, DK-2600 Glostrup, Denmark.

MANUEL J. JAYO DVM, PhD, Department of Comparative Medicine and the Comparative Medicine Clinical Research Center, Wake Forest University Medical Center, Winston-Salem, NC 27157, USA.

JYTTE JENSEN MD, Department of Endocrinology and Medicine, Herlev Hospital, University of Copenhagen, DK-2730 Herlev, Denmark.

ROBERT LINDSAY MB, ChB, PhD, FRCP, Chief of Internal Medicine, Helen Hayes Hospital, West Haverstraw, NY 10993-1195, USA; Professor of Clinical Medicine, Columbia University, College of Physicians and Surgeons, New York, USA.

L. JOSEPH MELTON, III MD, Professor of Epidemiology, Mayo Medical School; Head, Section of Clinical Epidemiology, Department of Health Sciences Research, Mayo Clinic, 200 First Street S.W., Rochester, MN 55905, USA.

KATHERINE MILLER BASS MD, Instructor, Department of Obstetrics and Gynecology, University of Maryland, 22 S. Greene Street, Baltimore, MD 21210, USA; Post-Doctoral Fellow, Department of Epidemiology, Johns Hopkins School of Hygiene and Public Health, 615 N. Wolfe Street, Baltimore, MD 21215, USA.

BENTE JUEL RIIS MD, Department of Clinical Chemistry, Glostrup Hospital, University of Copenhagen, DK-2600, Glostrup, Denmark.

ANNA N. A. TOSTESON ScD, Assistant Professor of Health Decision Sciences, Harvard School of Public Health; Instructor, Harvard Medical School, Beth Israel Hospital, Brigham and Women's Hospital, 75 Francis Street, Boston, MA 02115, USA.

MILTON C. WEINSTEIN PhD, Henry J. Kaiser Professor of Health Policy and Management, and Biostatistics, Harvard School of Public Health, 677 Huntington Avenue, Boston, MA 02115, USA.

J. KOUDY WILLIAMS DVM, Assistant Professor, CMCRC, Bowman Gray School of Medicine of Wake Forest University, 300 South Hawthorne Road, Winston-Salem, NC 27103, USA.

Table of contents

Foreword/C. CHRISTIANSEN   ix

1   Epidemiology of osteoporosis   785
L. J. MELTON III

2   Current techniques for bone mass measurement   807
C. HASSAGER & C. CHRISTIANSEN

3   What do we know about biochemical bone markers?   817
P. D. DELMAS

4   Biochemical markers—a new approach for identifying those at
risk of osteoporosis   831
B. J. RIIS

5   Why do oestrogens prevent bone loss?   837
R. LINDSAY

6   Hormone replacement therapy for established osteoporosis in
elderly women   853
C. CHRISTIANSEN

7   Do we have any alternatives to sex steroids in the prevention
and treatment of osteoporosis?   857
C. H. CHESNUT III

8   Effects of sex steroids on serum lipids and lipoproteins   867
J. JENSEN

9   Oestrogen therapy and cardiovascular disease: do the benefits
outweigh the risks?   889
T. L. BUSH & K. MILLER BASS

10   Effects of oestrogens and progestogens on coronary
atherosclerosis and osteoporosis of monkeys   915
M. R. ADAMS, J. K. WILLIAMS, T. B. CLARKSON & M. J. JAYO

11   Prevention of osteoporotic fractures: what we need to know   935
S. R. CUMMINGS

12   Cost-effectiveness of hormone replacement therapy after
the menopause   943
A. N. A. TOSTESON & M. C. WEINSTEIN

Index   961

PREVIOUS ISSUES

December 1989
Psychological Aspects of Obstetrics and Gynaecology
M. R. OATES

March 1990
Antenatal Care
M. HALL

June 1990
Medical Induction of Abortion
M. BYGDEMAN

September 1990
Induction of Ovulation
P. G. CROSIGNANI

December 1990
Computing and Decision Support in Obstetrics and Gynaecology
R. J. LILFORD

March 1991
Factors of Importance for Implantation
M. SEPPÄLÄ

June 1991
Diabetes in Pregnancy
J. N. OATS

September 1991
Human Reproduction: Current and Future Ethical Issues
W. A. W. WALTERS

FORTHCOMING ISSUES

March 1992
HIV Infection in Obstetrics and Gynaecology
F. D. JOHNSTONE

June 1992
Assisted Reproduction
L. HAMBERGER & M. WIKLAND

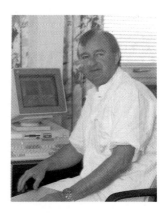

Foreword

An estimated 200 million people worldwide have osteoporosis, a disease characterized by a reduction in bone mass. This thinning of the bone tissue causes the skeleton (particularly the spine, wrist and hip) to become weak, brittle and susceptible to fracture. These fractures are one of the leading causes of morbidity and death in elderly people. The cost of osteoporosis is overwhelming and will constitute increasing burdens to the societies of Europe, the United States and Japan. Each year, 700 000 people suffer a hip fracture in these countries—about 20% of those people die within 6 months from complications—amounting to 140 000 people per year, or 16 people per hour!!! Half of the people affected never return to fully independent living.

In the past few years considerable progress has been made in how to predict women at risk, diagnose, prevent and treat this disabling disease. This raises the hope that soon osteoporosis may become 'a disease of the past'.

The mainstay of prevention and management of osteoporosis is hormone replacement therapy. This was the conclusion at all three international osteoporosis consensus development conferences held in 1984, 1987 and 1990. Oestrogen or oestrogen/progestogen replacement therapy is highly effective in preventing osteoporosis in women. It reduces bone resorption and halts postmenopausal bone loss. Epidemiological studies have shown a substantial reduction in hip, wrist and vertebral fractures in women whose replacement was begun within a few years of menopause. Observational studies have furthermore suggested that oestrogen therapy reduces the risk of cardiovascular disease substantially, with a similar effect on overall mortality.

There are still unanswered questions regarding hormone replacement therapy, such as the influence of combined oestrogen/progestogen on risk of cardiovascular disease and the effect of hormone replacement therapy on the risk of breast cancer.

Hormone replacement therapy prescribed for prevention of osteoporosis will often be a relatively long-term therapy. The object of this book is to give a comprehensive review of the potential benefits and risks that are especially associated with such a long-term treatment.

The field of osteoporosis is endowed with a large number of outstanding scientists. I am grateful that it has been possible to obtain contributions from such excellent experts who all have heavy workloads and too little leisure time. My thanks are thus also extended to all the families who have to live with an ever-working scientist. It is my hope that this book will increase the interest in osteoporosis.

CLAUS CHRISTIANSEN

1

Epidemiology of osteoporosis

L. JOSEPH MELTON III

Osteoporosis is important because it leads to skeletal fragility and an increased risk of fractures. This chapter will review the determinants of skeletal fragility, especially low bone mass, and will define the contributions to fracture risk made by low bone mass and trauma, particularly that related to falling. Risk factors for osteoporosis will then be explored, with a focus on those that result from insufficient bone mass in young adults and from subsequent bone loss due to the menopause in women, to ageing in both genders and to the various causes of secondary osteoporosis. This background is necessary for a proper understanding of alternatives for assessing and treating individual patients. Finally, the staggering burden of morbidity, mortality and cost that these fractures impose on the population will be recounted as a stimulus for greater clinical attention to this growing societal problem.

PATHOGENESIS OF OSTEOPOROSIS

Skeletal fragility

Bone strength is related to the material properties of bone tissue (bone quality) and to its structural arrangement (bone architecture). Bone is composed of a mineralized collagen matrix that is periodically renewed at specific foci, called bone multicellular units. Here, old bone is resorbed by osteoclasts and the resulting defect is then filled with new bone produced by osteoblasts (Parfitt, 1988). In adolescents, more bone is replaced than is removed so that bone mass increases (Figure 1). Following a period where the two processes are balanced, bone begins to diminish because bone formation does not keep pace with bone resorption. This loss of tissue produces the histological picture of osteoporosis (literally, 'porous bone'). The bone that is present is relatively normal in composition, in contrast to osteomalacia, where there is an excess of unmineralized collagen matrix. However, the quality of osteoporotic bone may be impaired, from a biomechanical point of view, by age-related slowing of the bone remodelling process. This leads both to the build-up of hypermineralized old bone, which is more fragile, and to the accumulation of skeletal microfractures (Melton et al, 1988).

Baillière's Clinical Obstetrics and Gynaecology—
Vol. 5, No. 4, December 1991
ISBN 0–7020–1548–2

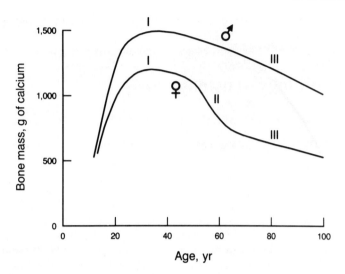

Figure 1. Changes in bone mass with ageing in men and women. Peak adult bone mass is reached in phase I before the start of net bone loss. Postmenopausal women and hypogonadal men have accelerated bone loss (phase II) superimposed upon the age-related bone loss (phase III), which occurs in both sexes. From Riggs & Melton (1992) with permission.

    While bone quality is important, the clinical consequences of osteoporosis relate mostly to the loss of bone tissue. With ageing, compact (or cortical) bone, which forms the shafts of the limbs and comprises up to 80% of the skeleton (Riggs and Melton, 1986), is lost from endosteal surfaces more rapidly than it is gained periosteally. This leads to a 30–50% reduction in the cortical thickness of these bones in women, with less dramatic reductions in men (Ruff and Hayes, 1982). Cortical thinning is partially compensated, biomechanically, by an age-related increase in diameter that improves resistance to bending and twisting (Melton et al, 1988). Since this may be sufficient to offset the bone loss, diaphyseal fractures generally reflect severe trauma and are not unduly common in osteoporotic patients.

    The remaining 20% of the skeleton is composed of cancellous (or trabecular) bone, which predominates in limb metaphyses and most of the axial skeleton. Cancellous bone loss leads to thinning and perforation of trabecular plates that form the internal supporting structure of the vertebrae, pelvis and other flat bones. Ultimately, some plates may be lost entirely. The thinning of vertical trabeculae and loss of interconnecting horizontal trabeculae, shown dramatically in Figure 2, results in a disproportionate loss of strength (Melton et al, 1988). For example, an age-related decrease of 45–50% in vertebral bone mass has been associated with a 75–89% reduction in compressive strength of the vertebral body (Mosekilde, 1989). The ability of the skeleton to withstand trauma is impaired as a consequence of these changes and, depending on the forces to which the bones are subjected, this may lead to fractures.

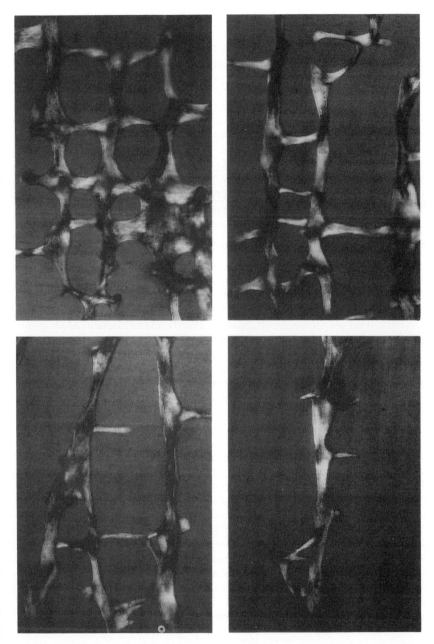

Figure 2. *Top left*: 50-year-old man with an almost 'perfect' continuous network of vertical and horizontal trabeculae. *Top right*: 58-year-old man with discernible thinning of the horizontal trabeculae and some loss of continuity. *Bottom left*: 76-year-old man with a continued thinning of the horizontal trabeculae and a wider separation of the vertical structures. *Bottom right*: 87-year-old woman with unsupported vertical trabeculae showing advanced breakdown of the whole network. From Mosekilde (1988) with permission.

Several important clinical principles derive from these biomechanical observations. First, there may be an irreversible component of bone loss. Available therapies are incapable of restoring structural elements of bone that have been completely lost. This dictates a strategy of early use of regimens which are able to slow or prevent bone loss. Second, treatments that increase bone mass may thicken existing bone structures rather than re-establish internal bone architecture. Consequently, fracture risk may not be reduced to the degree expected from observed increases in bone mineral. Finally, bone mass is not strictly synonymous with skeletal fragility. However, most of the ultimate strength of bone tissue is accounted for by bone mineral density (Melton et al, 1988), and the other main contributors to fragility (suboptimal bone geometry, impaired internal bone architecture, abnormalities of bone matrix or mineralization, and accumulation of micro-fractures) cannot be assessed non-invasively.

Relationship between osteoporosis and fractures

Population-based studies have shown increasing hip fracture incidence with declining bone mineral density in the proximal femur (Melton et al, 1986), rising Colles' fracture incidence with decreasing bone mass in the radius (Hui et al, 1988; Browner et al, 1989; Eastell et al, 1989) and increasing vertebral fracture incidence (Ross et al, 1988) and prevalence (Melton et al, 1989) with falling bone density in the lumbar spine. These gradients of risk are continuous, with no true biological threshold at which fractures begin (Figure 3). The overlap in values means that fracture patients cannot be clearly discriminated from age- and sex-matched controls. This is not necessary, however, since bone mineral measurements are not intended to diagnose fractures; instead, they predict the risk of future fractures, as shown by a number of prospective studies.

Although osteoporosis may not be recognized clinically until fractures occur, the processes that cause osteoporosis may have been progressing silently for decades. Prior to the onset of fractures, the only practical approach to diagnosis is on the basis of low bone mineral assessed in vivo. However, consensus has not been reached on the level of bone mineral that should spur clinical action (Melton and Wahner, 1989). Until a decision has been made on the 'fracture threshold' (really the treatment threshold) which defines the condition, there can be no precise answer to the question, 'How many people have osteoporosis?' By any definition, though, it is clear that a substantial portion of Caucasian women are affected. Rough estimates suggest that 20–25 million Americans are at increased risk of fracture by virtue of low bone mass (Peck et al, 1988), indicating that virtually every physician will be faced with managing this problem.

Risk factors for trauma

Because of their fragile skeletons, a substantial portion of elderly individuals, especially women, are susceptible to fractures. However, their likelihood of falling is also greater, rising annually from about one in five

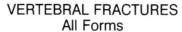

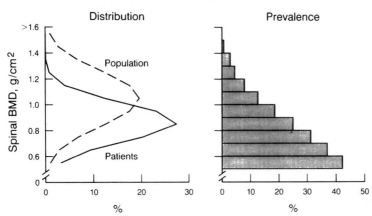

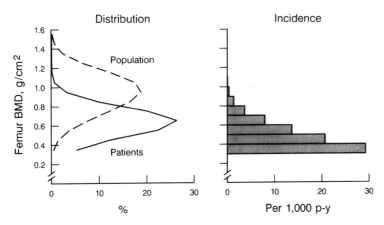

Figure 3. Distribution of spinal bone mineral density (BMD) of vertebral fracture patients and controls compared with vertebral fracture prevalence, and of hip BMD for intertrochanteric hip fracture patients and controls compared with hip fracture incidence among women from Rochester, Minnesota. p-y = person-years. From Melton et al (1990) with permission.

women 60–64 years old to one in three aged 80–84 years (Cummings and Nevitt, 1989). The pathophysiology of falling is poorly understood and, in a specific patient, usually results from a complex interaction of several factors (Melton, 1988). Descriptive studies indicate that half or more of the falls among elderly persons are associated with organic dysfunction such as diminished postural control, gait changes, muscular weakness, decreased reflexes or poor vision. The proportion of persons with one or more of these problems increases with age, and the risk of falling is directly correlated with the number of conditions present (Tinetti et al, 1988).

Specific diseases play a role in some falls (Melton, 1988). Most often mentioned are parkinsonism, stroke or hemiplegia, cardiac rhythm or output defects, pneumonia, arthritis, and alcoholism. 'Drop attacks', postulated to result from disturbances in blood flow to brain stem postural centres, may cause an additional 10–20% of falls among elderly persons. Iatrogenic problems include excessive use of sedatives and overtreatment of hypertension. Environmental factors, like slippery surfaces, loose rugs and light cords, may be responsible for a third to a half of all falls, but these operate in the context of the physiological abnormalities noted above. The risk of falling may be greater at night, but most falls occur during daylight hours when older people are most active.

It is important to note, however, that most falls do not result in an injury, even among the elderly. Only 5–6% of falls lead to a fracture and only 1% lead to a hip fracture (Gibson, 1987). Thus, additional risk factors are needed to account for the full spectrum of fall outcomes. These are likely to relate to the mechanics of falling (Melton and Riggs, 1985). Recent data indicate, for example, that the orientation of the fall is a potentially dominant factor. In one study of nursing home residents, the relative risk of a hip fracture was increased over 13-fold with a fall on the hip or side of the leg (Hayes et al, 1991). While the impact force was somewhat reduced by the amount of soft tissue padding over the hip, the potential energy in a fall directly on the hip was sufficient to fracture the femurs of most elderly individuals. Thus, prevention of the clinical manifestations of osteoporosis will depend in large part on reducing the frequency and severity of falls.

RISK FACTORS FOR OSTEOPOROSIS

Because the risk factors for falling are difficult to correct, it is prudent to maximize bone mass throughout life. Indeed, this is the only intervention that can be undertaken in young and middle-aged individuals with the hope of preventing fractures later. A number of approaches have been developed (see Chapters 6 and 11), but it is not yet certain how they might best be targeted at high-risk individuals in the population. Alternatives include screening potential candidates for therapy with bone mineral measurements (see Chapter 2), with biochemical markers of bone metabolism (see Chapter 3), with risk factor scores, or with some combination of these. The development of risk factor profiles is complicated by the diverse influences on bone mass. Thus, a person's risk of osteoporosis is determined by the peak bone mass achieved in young adulthood as well as by the subsequent rate of bone loss (Figure 4). This bone loss results from age-related factors that occur universally in the population and account for slow bone loss over life in both sexes, from an accelerated phase of bone loss associated with the menopause in women and hypogonadism in some men, and from medical and surgical conditions that produce 'secondary' osteoporosis (Riggs and Melton, 1986).

PATHOGENESIS OF OSTEOPOROSIS
Model

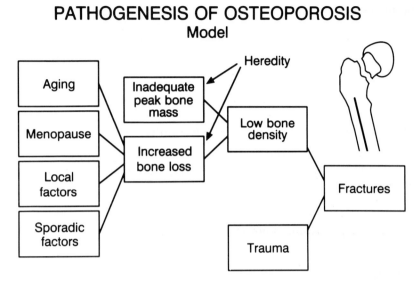

Figure 4. Conceptual model of the pathogenesis of fractures related to osteoporosis. Modified from Riggs (1988).

A person's bone mass is the net result of these factors, the relative importance of which may vary from one individual to another.

Peak bone mass

The smaller the bone mass accumulated during skeletal growth and consolidation, the greater is the risk of fractures later in life when bone loss ensues. Little is known of the factors that influence peak bone mass, although a genetic component is obvious (Kelly et al, 1990). Thus, race and gender differences in the incidence of osteoporosis and fractures are explained in part by the heritability of skeletal size (Figure 5). Bone mass is greatest in those of African heritage, who have the lowest fracture rates, and is least in Caucasian women of Northern European extraction, who have the highest fracture rates (Melton, 1991). Within each ethnic group, men have a greater mass, and lower fracture rates, than women.

However, these generalizations are valid only for groups; many white women never experience a hip fracture, for example, while some black men do. Consequently, it is important to delineate the factors that determine peak bone mass in the individual. It is generally appreciated that sex steroids and growth hormones modulate normal development of the skeleton. Studies have also shown a positive correlation between peak bone mass and calcium intake (Sowers et al, 1985a), and the secular trend of increasing skeletal size is credited to dietary changes. Moderate exercise also increases bone mass in the young (Drinkwater et al, 1990), and there is growing evidence that diet and activity are synergistic (Kanders et al, 1988). On the other hand, exercise regimens so extreme as to induce amenorrhoea cause

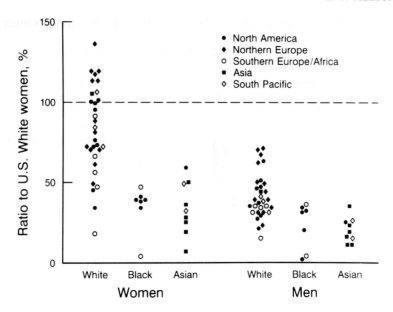

Figure 5. Hip fracture incidence as a ratio of the rates observed to those expected for United States white women of the same age. From Melton (1991) with permission.

bone loss (Drinkwater et al, 1990), as does anorexia nervosa (Rigotti et al, 1991). The effects of other risk factors, such as pregnancy, lactation and oral contraceptive use, are inconsistent and generally weak (L. J. Melton, S. L. Cedel, H. W. Wahner et al, unpublished data), although there is recent interest in the influence of more subtle menstrual irregularities.

Other than promote good nutrition and adequate exercise, the clinician can do little to enhance peak bone mass in adolescents and young adults, although ongoing research in this area may lead to more focused interventions in the future. Nonetheless, it is necessary to recognize that initial bone mass is an important determinant of bone mass later in life; it has been estimated that bone mass at age 70 years is influenced about equally by peak bone mass and subsequent bone loss (Hui et al, 1990). Thus, individuals with marginal peak bone mass represent a high risk group for the clinician concerned about menopausal or age-related bone loss.

Age-related bone loss

With ageing, bone mass gradually diminishes (Figure 1). The determinants of this slow form of bone loss are not precisely known, but calcium metabolism may be disturbed by dysfunction in a number of organ systems. For example, an age-related loss of kidney tissue (with its enzyme, 25-hydroxyvitamin D_1 α-hydroxylase) slows conversion of 25-hydroxyvitamin D to the active metabolite, 1,25-dihydroxyvitamin D (Riggs and Melton,

1992). This reduces active calcium absorption from the gut, as does intestinal resistance to vitamin D caused possibly by an age-related decrease in vitamin D receptors (Eastell et al, 1991). Inadequate calcium absorption leads, in turn, to secondary hyperparathyroidism. The resulting increase in the rate of bone turnover causes bone loss because of the uncoupling of bone formation from bone resorption. This is the proposed pathogenesis of type II (or age-related) osteoporosis (Table 1), which commonly occurs in elderly women and men and is characterized by loss of both compact and cancellous bone at a rate similar to that in the general population (Riggs and Melton, 1986). Type II osteoporosis is linked to hip fractures and to fractures of the proximal humerus, pelvis and distal femur, among others (Melton, 1988).

Table 1. Comparison of two types of involutional osteoporosis. From Riggs and Melton (1986) with permission.

	Type I	Type II
Age (years)	51–75	>70
Sex ratio (female:male)	6:1	2:1
Type of bone loss	Mainly cancellous	Cancellous and compact
Rate of bone loss	Accelerated	Not accelerated
Fracture sites	Vertebrae (crush) and distal radius	Vertebrae (wedge) and hip
Parathyroid function	Decreased	Increased
Calcium absorption	Decreased	Decreased
Metabolism of 25-OH-D to 1,25(OH)$_2$D	Secondary decrease	Primary decrease
Main causes	Factors related to menopause	Factors related to ageing

25-OH-D = 25-hydroxyvitamin D; 1,25(OH)$_2$D = dihydroxyvitamin D.

The decline in active calcium absorption with ageing can be overcome by increasing calcium intake in order to augment passive calcium absorption. The calcium intake needed to accomplish this is controversial. Population studies have not demonstrated a strong relationship between calcium intake and bone loss or fractures (Kanis and Passmore, 1989), while clinical trials have generally found little effect on spinal bone loss and only a modest effect on appendicular bone loss of calcium supplementation shortly after the menopause (Cumming, 1990). However, the results of recent clinical trials in older women are more encouraging (Dawson-Hughes et al, 1990), and it would seem prudent to assure at least the minimum recommended levels of calcium intake at all ages. Likewise, vitamin D intake should be sufficient to overcome age-related decreases in vitamin D metabolism (Riggs and Melton, 1992). There is as yet no evidence, however, that calcium and/or vitamin D supplementation will reduce the risk of age-related fractures or provide a viable alternative to oestrogen replacement therapy in perimenopausal women.

Age-related bone loss could also relate to declining physical activity and fitness (Pocock et al, 1989). In one well-known study, bone mineral content in the lumbar spine decreased about 0.9% per week (one year's worth!) in a group of hospitalized adults on complete bed rest (Krølner and Toft, 1983). Conversely, increased activity might help maintain bone mass and prevent osteoporosis. A protective effect of exercise has been hypothesized to explain the lower prevalence of osteoporosis among women of Asian or African heritage (Melton, 1991). For example, compared with Johannesburg whites, Bantu women show little bone loss between 30 and 50 years of age; this has been attributed to declining physical activity in middle-aged whites that is not seen in the Bantu, who continue to perform hard physical labour (Solomon, 1979). Short-term clinical trials suggest that exercise programmes can also augment bone mass, but the improvements are inconsistent and it is not certain whether any gains are maintained or lead to a reduction in fractures (Block et al, 1989).

Menopausal bone loss

Oestrogen deficiency is an important cause of bone loss and subsequent fractures in women. While all women experience menopause, a smaller proportion of them develop the distal forearm fractures and postmenopausal vertebral fractures that are hypothesized to be manifestations of type I (postmenopausal) osteoporosis (Riggs and Melton, 1986). As delineated in Table 1, oestrogen deficiency leads to increased bone turnover (there is an increase in bone formation but an even greater increase in bone resorption). Due to the larger surface area involved, trabecular and endocortical bone are disproportionately affected by this accelerated bone loss (Parfitt, 1988), which can be prevented by oestrogen replacement therapy (see Chapter 6). In the absence of such therapy, bone appears to become more sensitive to the effects of parathyroid hormone (Kotowicz et al, 1990), but additional causal factors must be present and interact with oestrogen deficiency to determine individual susceptibility. Possibilities include increased local production of interleukin 1 or another factor that increases bone resorption, prolongation of the accelerated phase of bone loss, low bone mass at the inception of menopause, or some combination of these (Riggs and Melton, 1986).

The accelerated phase of bone loss in perimenopausal women is superimposed upon the slower, age-related bone loss (Riggs and Melton, 1986), and explains in part the two-fold higher incidence of fractures among women than men later in life (Melton, 1988). However, an important role for menopause has not been found in all epidemiological studies (Seeman et al, 1988). Discrepancies are probably accounted for by this additive effect. Age at menopause is a better determinant of bone mass in the midst of the accelerated phase, while chronological age is more closely correlated with bone mass later in life. This accords with data showing that bone mass decreases as a logarithmic function of years since the menopause (Gallagher et al, 1987). Clinically, this suggests that the age at menopause will have little utility as a risk factor among elderly women, but could be important among younger women who have had an early menopause. Hypogonadism also occurs in a small proportion of men and may lead to bone loss (Finkelstein et al, 1987) and fractures (Seeman et al, 1983).

Secondary osteoporosis

Bone loss is exacerbated by specific conditions that occur sporadically in the population (Riggs and Melton, 1986). Some are diseases like acromegaly, Cushing's disease and multiple myeloma, which are sufficiently uncommon that they contribute little to the community burden of osteoporosis. Others, such as hyperthyroidism, hyperparathyroidism and corticosteroid use are more important (Melton and Riggs, 1988). Glucocorticoids, for example, produce rapid bone loss through enhancement of bone resorption and inhibition of bone formation and lead to fractures in a substantial proportion of patients on long-term treatment (Lukert and Raisz, 1990). Other putative causes of secondary osteoporosis are only indirectly related to bone loss and fractures. The adverse effects of rheumatoid arthritis and stroke, for example, are mostly due to disuse osteoporosis (Melton and Riggs, 1988). In still other instances, the primary pathophysiology is uncertain. Chronic obstructive lung disease, for example, may be associated with metabolic abnormalities, with smoking and ethanol use which have toxic effects on bone (Baron, 1984; Turner et al, 1987), with inactivity, and with corticosteroid use. While medical or surgical conditions may be a major cause of osteoporosis in some individuals, any resulting bone loss is additive to age-related and menopausal bone loss (Riggs and Melton, 1986). Thus, vertebral fractures are more likely to occur in postmenopausal women taking corticosteroids than in premenopausal women on the same regimen (Dyckman et al, 1985). Altogether, one or more of the causes of secondary osteoporosis is present in up to 20% of women and 40% of men with vertebral or hip fractures (Melton and Riggs, 1988).

Conversely, thiazide diuretic therapy appears to be protective against bone loss and fractures (Wasnich et al, 1983; Ray et al, 1989; Felson et al, 1991), possibly as a result of reduced urinary calcium excretion. Thiazide therapy is not innocuous, however, and no regimen for its use in preventing osteoporosis has yet been developed. Obesity exerts a protective effect through increased skeletal loading and enhanced endogenous oestrogen production (Johnston et al, 1985). If the latter mechanism were predominant, obesity and oestrogen replacement therapy might act through a final common pathway mediated by a direct oestrogen effect on bone cells (Eriksen et al, 1988).

CLINICAL USE OF RISK FACTORS

Bone mass estimation

There has been great interest in predicting bone mass using the various risk factors enumerated above, but this has proven to be difficult. Most studies have been relatively small, and various investigators have emphasized different sets of risk factors or associated them with different measures of bone mass. For example, age, height, weight and serum oestrogen concentration accounted for only 22–37% of the variability in bone mineral at the os calcis and forearm in 43–80-year-old Hawaiian women of Japanese ancestry

(Yano et al, 1984), while age, humeral muscle area, use of oestrogen replacement therapy, thiazides or vitamin D, and calcium intake over 800 mg/day explained 40% of the variance in bone mineral content of the mid-radius in a population-based study of 324 Iowa women aged 55–80 years (Sowers et al, 1985b). In a study of perimenopausal women (e.g. a population for whom oestrogen therapy would be considered), height, weight, cigarette smoking, calcium intake and urinary calcium-creatinine ratio accounted for between 17% (femoral neck) and 47% (mid-radius) of the variability in bone mineral measurements (Slemenda et al, 1990). This combination of variables correctly classified about two-thirds of the women whose bone mass was in the lowest tertile (Figure 6). Studies in series of volunteers have found similar results (Johnston et al, 1989). Together, these results demonstrate that the various risk factors so far identified, while statistically significant, account for only about half of the variability in bone mass.

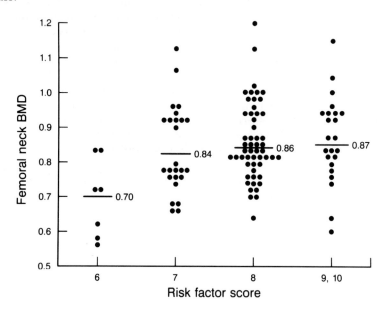

Figure 6. Observed femoral neck bone mineral density (BMD) plotted against risk factor score. From Slemenda et al (1990) with permission.

Fracture prediction

Efforts to predict fractures directly from risk factor scores have been even less successful. For example, 90% of one group of 704 postmenopausal women had at least four of the putative risk factors for vertebral fractures; no factor alone or in combination accurately predicted the occurrence of a new vertebral fracture over the duration of follow-up (Wasnich et al, 1987). More recently, a risk factor score (age, lactation, nulliparity, metacarpal index, height and age at menarche) was able to discriminate among 1014

Dutch women aged 45–64 years who did and did not incur subsequent fractures over 9 years of follow-up; unfortunately, the specificity (83–84%) and, especially, the sensitivity (37–48%) were low (van Hemert et al, 1990). Thus, no set of risk factors has been shown to predict bone mass or fractures with sufficient accuracy for application to individual patient care. Nonetheless, efforts must continue to identify the patients at greatest risk of subsequent fractures, and numerous epidemiological studies now underway should lead to better clinical approaches to this problem in the future.

IMPACT OF OSTEOPOROTIC FRACTURES

Morbidity

The fractures caused by osteoporosis have been identified by epidemiological criteria to include those that increase dramatically in incidence with ageing, are more frequent in women than men, and occur with minimal or moderate trauma at sites containing disproportionate amounts of cancellous bone. Thus, fractures of the hip, vertebrae and distal forearm have been designated as age-related fractures (Figure 7), along with some pelvic, proximal humerus and proximal tibia fractures (Melton, 1988). However, the introduction of bone absorptiometry has allowed this relationship to be evaluated directly, and it is now recognized that most fractures in the elderly are due, in part, to low bone mass (Seeley et al, 1990). Thus, the clinical horizon must be broadened, even though available data are mostly limited to the sites traditionally associated with osteoporosis.

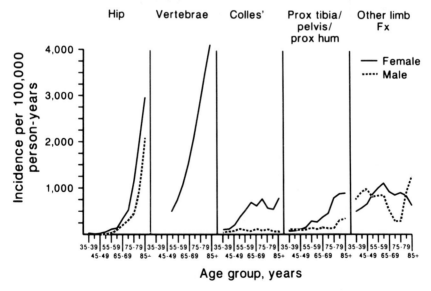

Figure 7. Age- and sex-specific incidence rates for various fractures among residents of Rochester, Minnesota. Prox = proximal; hum = humerus; Fx = fractures. From Melton and Cummings (1987) with permission.

Table 2. Impact of fractures in the United States.

	Hip fracture	Wrist fracture	Spine fracture
Excess mortality	12%	None	None?
Morbidity:			
Lifetime risk	15% female;	15% female;	35% female;
	5% male	2% male	? male
Cases per year	~250 000	~240 000	~500 000
Disability	+++	+	++
Cost	All fracture sites combined = $18 billion (1984)		

(From Osteoporosis. In Berg RL & Cassells JS (eds) *The Second Fifty Years: Promoting Health and Preventing Disability*, pp 76–100. Washington: National Academy Press.)

Were it not for the fractures, osteoporosis would have little practical significance. Unfortunately, such fractures are common, and their medical and social consequences make osteoporosis an enormous public health problem (Table 2). It has been estimated that there may be a quarter of a million hip fractures and wrist fractures and perhaps twice that number of vertebral fractures in the United States each year (Melton, 1988). The significance of these numbers is better grasped by noting that the lifetime risk of a hip fracture—15% in white women and 5% in men (Cummings et al, 1985)—is equivalent to the combined lifetime risk of developing breast, uterine or ovarian cancer in women and about the same as the lifetime risk of prostate cancer in men. The lifetime risk of a Colles' fracture from age 50 years onward is also 15% in women and a little over 2% in white men (Cummings et al, 1985). The skeletal site most affected by osteoporosis, however, is the spine. The prevalence of vertebral fractures among 70-year-old Danish women was 21% (Jensen et al, 1982). Altogether, almost a third of women aged 65 years and over will have one or more vertebral fractures if all forms are included (Melton et al, 1989). The condition is so ubiquitous, then, that almost every clinician will be faced with the problem in his or her own patients.

Mortality

Hip fractures lead to an overall 5–20% reduction in expected survival (Cummings et al, 1985). The excess mortality may be seen for up to 6 months following the fracture and varies with age and gender. For example, about 90% of hip fracture victims under 75 years of age are still alive at 1 year (92% of expected), compared with only 73% (83% of expected) of those aged 75 years and over at the time of fracture (Melton, 1988). Despite their greater average age at the time of the fracture, survival is better among women, 83% of whom are still alive 1 year later compared with only 63% of men. In contrast, wrist fractures cause no increase in mortality (Melton, 1988). There is no published information concerning the influence of vertebral fractures on life expectancy. Mortality following hip fracture is mediated primarily by coexisting serious illnesses (Magaziner et al, 1989), which probably also explain the observation that death rates are increased among women with low bone mass (Browner et al, 1990). As alarming as these data may be, however, the adverse consequences of osteoporosis relate less to mortality than to the long-term disability that may result.

Disability

Many hip fracture patients are non-ambulatory even before the fracture. Of those able to walk before sustaining a hip fracture, however, half cannot walk independently afterward (Miller, 1978). The ability of such patients to care for themselves is compromised, and poor ambulation is one of the predictors of nursing home admission (Ceder et al, 1980; Bonar et al, 1990). In addition, hip fracture survivors often develop other complications, such as pressure sores, pneumonia and urinary tract infections, and may become severely depressed (Mossey et al, 1989). Ultimately, up to a third of hip fracture victims may become totally dependent (Jensen and Bagger, 1982), and the risk of institutionalization is great, with over 60 000 nursing home admissions attributed to hip fractures annually in the United States (Phillips et al, 1988).

Distal forearm fractures have generally been considered free of long-term disability, but recent reviews show that persistent pain, loss of function, neuropathies and post-traumatic arthritis are quite common (de Bruijn, 1987). Collapse fractures of the vertebrae may lead to progressive loss of height, kyphosis, postural changes and persistent pain that interferes with the activities of daily living (Sinaki, 1988). Because only a minority of vertebral fracture patients are medically attended, neither acute nor chronic disabilities have ever been assessed in a systematic way.

Cost

The total cost of fractures may be as much as $18 billion per year in the United States, and osteoporosis accounts for at least a third of this (Holbrook et al, 1984), estimated most recently at $7–10 billion annually (Peck et al, 1988). Because most of these fractures are in elderly individuals, the important determinants of cost are inpatient and outpatient medical services and nursing home care. This included an estimated 322 000 hospitalizations and almost 4 million hospital days for women 45 years old and over in the United States in 1986, where osteoporosis-related conditions were the primary cause of admission; more than half of the total was for hip fractures (Phillips et al, 1988). Osteoporosis was a contributing cause of admission in an additional 170 000 hospitalizations for an extra 290 000 hospital days. In women of this age, there were 2.3 million physician visits for osteoporosis in 1986. At each visit, a third of the women needed an X-ray, a fourth required physiotherapy, and most received a prescribed medication for the condition. There were also an estimated 83 000 nursing home stays for osteoporosis-related causes in the United States in 1986, with an average duration of stay of 1 year. Altogether, these direct costs of osteoporosis totalled $5.2 billion for women alone (Phillips et al, 1988). In England, hip fracture patients were estimated to be occupying one-fifth of all orthopaedic beds, at a direct cost in England and Wales of £160 million per year in 1988 (Hoffenberg et al,

1989). In France, there are an estimated 40 000–65 000 vertebral fractures, 56 000 hip fractures and 35 000 distal forearm fractures annually; the hip and wrist fractures together are estimated to cost 3.7 billion French francs each year (Levy, 1989). Analogous figures from almost every Western country are a source of great concern to governmental leaders.

Prospects for the future

Unfortunately, costs can only rise in the future because the elderly population is growing rapidly throughout the world. In the United States, for example, the actual number of individuals aged 65 years and over will increase from 30 to 67 million between 1988 and 2050. Since the incidence of osteoporosis-related fractures rises with age, demographic changes alone will eventually result in a doubling or tripling of the number of hip fractures seen each year, with increases for the other fracture sites as well. It is projected that in only 30 years' time there could be almost 350 000 hip fractures in the United States each year, at an annual cost estimated to be between \$31 and \$62 billion (Cummings et al, 1990). Hip fractures might increase in the United Kingdom from 46 000 in 1985 to 60 000 in 2016 (Hoffenberg et al, 1989), and in Australia from 10 150 in 1986 to 18 550 in 2011 (Lord and Sinnett, 1986). Health authorities in Finland expect a 38% increase in the number of hip fractures between 1983 and 2010 and a 71% increase in the hospital bed-days needed to care for these patients (Simonen, 1988). This alarming situation could be made even worse by rising fracture incidence rates. Observations in many countries are generally consistent with a widespread increase in hip fracture incidence among both men and

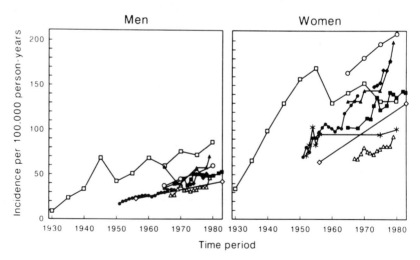

Figure 8. Incidence of hip fractures over time as reported from various studies □—□ Rochester, Minnesota; ■—■ United States: ◇—◇ Oxford, England; ◆—◆ Funen County, Denmark; △—△ Holland; ▲—▲ Göteborg, Sweden; ○—○ Uppsala, Sweden; ●—● New Zealand; ★—★ Dundee, Scotland. From Melton et al (1987) with permission.

women, even after adjustment for the growth in the elderly population (Figure 8). While some studies hint that the rate of rise may now be slowing (Melton, 1990), the message is clear that unless therapeutic or, preferably, prophylactic interventions are implemented on a large scale, the economic and social costs of osteoporosis will continue to grow.

SUMMARY

A variety of pathophysiological mechanisms lead to bone loss. The decreased bone mass results in an increased risk of fractures, which are the sole clinical manifestation of osteoporosis. Thus, it is not surprising that osteoporosis should be seen as a complex, multifactorial chronic disease that may progress silently for decades until characteristic fractures result late in life. Because there are no symptoms until fractures occur, relatively few people are diagnosed in time for effective therapy to be administered. Consequently, a large number of individuals experience the pain, expense, disability and decreased quality of life caused by these age-related fractures. This important public health problem will worsen in the future as the population ages, unless suitable interventions can be devised. Preventing excessive bone loss is the only action that can be taken now to reduce fractures in the future, and the following chapters describe clinical strategies for identifying and treating those believed to be at greatest risk.

Acknowledgements

I would like to thank Mrs Yvonne Weeldreyer for help in preparing the manuscript.
    This work was supported in part by research grant AR-27065 from the National Institutes of Health, US Public Health Service.

REFERENCES

Baron JA (1984) Smoking and estrogen-related disease. *American Journal of Epidemiology* **119:** 9–22.
Block JE, Smith R, Friedlander A & Genant HK (1989) Preventing osteoporosis with exercise: a review with emphasis on methodology. *Medical Hypotheses* **30:** 9–19.
Bonar SK, Tinetti ME, Speechley M & Cooney LM (1990) Factors associated with short- versus long-term skilled nursing facility placement among community-living hip fracture patients. *Journal of the American Geriatrics Society* **38:** 1139–1144.
Browner WS, Cummings SR, Genant HK et al for the Study of Osteoporotic Fractures Research Group (1989) Bone mineral density and fractures of the wrist and humerus in elderly women: A prospective study. *Journal of Bone and Mineral Research* **4(supplement 1):** S171.
Browner WS, Seeley DG, Black D et al and the Study of Osteoporotic Fractures Research Group, Universities of California (San Francisco), Pittsburgh, Maryland, Minnesota, and the Kaiser Permanente Center for Health Research, Portland, Oregon, USA (1990) The association between bone mineral density and mortality in elderly women. In Christiansen C & Overgaard K (eds) *Osteoporosis 1990*, vol. 1, pp 71–72. Copenhagen: Osteopress ApS.

Ceder L, Thorngren K-G & Wallden B (1980) Prognostic indicators and early home rehabilitation in elderly patients with hip fractures. *Clinical Orthopaedics and Related Research* **152:** 173–184.

Cummings RG (1990) Calcium intake and bone mass: A quantitative review of the evidence. *Calcified Tissue International* **47:** 194–201.

Cummings SR & Nevitt MC (1989) Epidemiology of hip fractures and falls. In Kleerekoper M & Krane SM (eds) *Clinical Disorders of Bone and Mineral Metabolism*, pp 231–236. New York: Mary Ann Liebert.

Cummings SR, Kelsey JL, Nevitt MC & O'Dowd KJ (1985) Epidemiology of osteoporosis and osteoporotic fractures. *Epidemiologic Reviews* **7:** 178–208.

Cummings SR, Rubin SM & Black D (1990) The future of hip fractures in the United States: Numbers, costs, and potential effects of postmenopausal estrogen. *Clinical Orthopaedics and Related Research* **252:** 163–166.

Dawson-Hughes B, Dallal GE, Krall EA et al (1990) A controlled trial of the effect of calcium supplementation on bone density in postmenopausal women. *New England Journal of Medicine* **323:** 878–883.

de Bruijn HP (1987) The Colles fracture, review of literature. *Acta Orthopaedica Scandinavica* **58(supplement 223):** 7–25.

Drinkwater BL, Bruemner B & Chestnut CH (1990) Menstrual history as a determinant of current bone density in young athletes. *Journal of the American Medical Association* **263:** 545–548.

Dyckman TR, Gluck OS, Murphy WA, Hahn TJ & Hahn BH (1985) Evaluation of factors associated with glucocorticoid-induced osteopenia in patients with rheumatic diseases. *Arthritis and Rheumatism* **28:** 361–368.

Eastell R, Riggs BL, Wahner HW et al (1989) Colles' fracture and bone density of the ultradistal radius. *Journal of Bone and Mineral Research* **4:** 607–613.

Eastell R, Yergey AL, Vieira NE et al (1991) Interrelationship among vitamin D metabolism, true calcium absorption, parathyroid function, and age in women: evidence of an age-related intestinal resistance to 1,25-dihydroxyvitamin D action. *Journal of Bone and Mineral Research* **6:** 125–132.

Eriksen EF, Colvard DS, Berg NJ et al (1988) Evidence of estrogen receptors in normal human osteoblast-like cells. *Science* **241:** 84–86.

Felson DT, Sloutskis D, Anderson JJ, Anthony JM & Kiel DP (1991) Thiazide diuretics and the risk of hip fracture: Results from the Framingham study. *Journal of the American Medical Association* **265:** 370–373.

Finkelstein JS, Klibanski A, Neer RM et al (1987) Osteoporosis in men with idiopathic hypogonadotropic hypogonadism. *Annals of Internal Medicine* **106:** 354–361.

Gallagher JC, Goldar D & Moy A (1987) Total bone calcium in normal women: Effect of age and menopause status. *Journal of Bone and Mineral Research* **2:** 491–496.

Gibson MJ (1987) The prevention of falls in later life. *Danish Medical Bulletin* **34(supplement 4):** 1–24.

Hayes WC, Piazza SJ & Zysset PK (1991) Biomechanics of fracture risk prediction of the hip and spine by quantitative computed tomography. *Radiologic Clinics of North America* **29:** 1–18.

Hoffenberg R, James OFW, Brocklehurst JC et al (1989) Fractured neck of femur: Prevention and management. Summary and recommendations of a report of the Royal College of Physicians. *Journal of the Royal College of Physicians of London* **23:** 8–12.

Holbrook TL, Grazier K, Kelsey JL & Stauffer RN (1984) *The Frequency of Occurrence, Impact and Cost of Selected Musculoskeletal Conditions in the United States*, 187 pp. Chicago: American Academy of Orthopedic Surgeons.

Hui SL, Slemenda CW & Johnston CC Jr (1988) Age and bone mass as predictors of fracture in a prospective study. *Journal of Clinical Investigation* **81:** 1804–1809.

Hui SL, Slemenda CW & Johnston CC Jr (1990) The contribution of bone loss to postmenopausal osteoporosis. *Osteoporosis International* **1:** 30–34.

Jensen GF, Christiansen C, Boesen J, Hegedüs V & Transbøl I (1982) Epidemiology of postmenopausal spinal and long bone fractures: A unifying approach to postmenopausal osteoporosis. *Clinical Orthopaedics and Related Research* **166:** 75–81.

Jensen JS & Bagger J (1982) Long-term social prognosis after hip fractures. *Acta Orthopaedica Scandinavica* **53:** 97–101.

Johnston CC Jr, Hui SL & Longcope C (1985) Bone mass and sex steroid concentrations in postmenopausal Caucasian diabetics. *Metabolism: Clinical and Experimental* **34:** 544–550.

Johnston CC Jr, Melton LJ, Lindsay R & Eddy DM (1989) Clinical indications for bone mass measurements: A report from the Scientific Advisory Board of the National Osteoporosis Foundation. *Journal of Bone and Mineral Research* **4(supplement 2):** 1–28.

Kanders B, Dempster DW & Lindsay R (1988) Interaction of calcium nutrition and physical activity on bone mass in young women. *Journal of Bone and Mineral Research* **3:** 145–149.

Kanis JA & Passmore R (1989) Calcium supplementation of the diet—II: Not justified by present evidence. *British Medical Journal* **298:** 205–208.

Kelly PJ, Eisman JA & Sambrook PN (1990) Interaction of genetic and environmental influences on peak bone density. *Osteoporosis International* **1:** 56–60.

Kotowicz MA, Klee GG, Kao PC et al (1990) Relationship between serum intact parathyroid hormone concentrations and bone remodeling in type I osteoporosis: Evidence that skeletal sensitivity is increased. *Osteoporosis International* **1:** 14–22.

Krølner B & Toft B (1983) Vertebral bone loss: An unheeded side effect of therapeutic bed rest. *Clinical Science* **64:** 537–540.

Levy E (1989) Cost analysis of oestoporosis related to untreated menopause. *Clinical Rheumatology* **8(supplement 2):** 76–82.

Lord SR & Sinnett PF (1986) Femoral neck fractures: Admissions, bed use, outcome and projections. *Medical Journal of Australia* **145:** 493–496.

Lukert BP & Raisz LG (1990) Glucocorticoid-induced osteoporosis: Pathogenesis and management. *Annals of Internal Medicine* **112:** 352–364.

Magaziner J, Simonsick EM, Kashner TM, Hebel JR & Kenzora JE (1989) Survival experience of aged hip fracture patients. *American Journal of Public Health* **79:** 274–278.

Melton LJ III (1988) Epidemiology of fractures. In Riggs BL & Melton LJ III (eds) *Osteoporosis: Etiology, Diagnosis, and Management*, pp 133–154. New York: Raven Press.

Melton LJ III (1990) Epidemiology of fractures in North America. In Christiansen C & Overgaard K (eds) *Osteoporosis 1990*, vol. 1, pp 36–41. Copenhagen: Osteopress.

Melton LJ (1991) Differing patterns of osteoporosis across the world. *Excerpta Medica* (in press).

Melton LJ III & Cummings SR (1987) Heterogeneity of age-related fractures: Implications for epidemiology. *Bone and Mineral* **2:** 321–331.

Melton LJ III & Riggs BL (1985) Risk factors for injury after a fall. *Clinics in Geriatric Medicine* **1:** 525–539.

Melton LJ III & Riggs BL (1988) Clinical spectrum. In Riggs BL & Melton LJ III (eds) *Osteoporosis: Etiology, Diagnosis, and Management*, pp 155–179. New York: Raven Press.

Melton LJ III & Wahner HW (1989) Defining osteoporosis. *Calcified Tissue International* **45:** 263–264.

Melton LJ III, Wahner HW, Richelson LS, O'Fallon WM & Riggs BL (1986) Osteoporosis and the risk of hip fracture. *American Journal of Epidemiology* **124:** 254–261.

Melton LJ, O'Fallon WM & Riggs BL (1987) Secular trends in the incidence of hip fractures. *Calcified Tissue International* **41:** 57.

Melton LJ III, Chao EYS & Lane J (1988) Biomechanical aspects of fractures. In Riggs BL & Melton LJ III (eds) *Osteoporosis: Etiology, Diagnosis, and Management*, pp 111–131. New York: Raven Press.

Melton LJ, Kan SH, Frye MA et al (1989) Epidemiology of vertebral fractures in women. *American Journal of Epidemiology* **129:** 1000–1011.

Melton LJ, Eddy DM & Johnston CC (1990) Screening for osteoporosis. *Annals of Internal Medicine* **112:** 516–528.

Miller CW (1978) Survival and ambulation following hip fracture. *Journal of Bone and Joint Surgery* **60A:** 930–934.

Mosekilde Li (1988) Age-related changes in vertebral trabecular bone architecture—assessed by a new method. *Bone* **9:** 247–250.

Mosekilde Li (1989) Sex differences in age-related loss of vertebral trabecular bone mass and structure—biomechanical consequences. *Bone* **10:** 425–432.

Mossey JM, Mutran E, Knott K & Craik R (1989) Determinants of recovery 12 months after hip fracture: The importance of psychosocial factors. *American Journal of Public Health* **79:** 279–286.

Parfitt AM (1988) Bone remodeling: Relationship to the amount and structure of bone, and the pathogenesis and prevention of fractures. In Riggs BL & Melton LJ III (eds) *Osteoporosis: Etiology, Diagnosis, and Management*, pp 45–93. New York. Raven Press.

Peck WA, Riggs BL, Bell NH et al (1988) Research directions in osteoporosis. *American Journal of Medicine* **84:** 275–282.

Phillips S, Fox N, Jacobs J & Wright WE (1988) The direct medical costs of osteoporosis for American women aged 45 and older, 1986. *Bone* **9:** 271–279.

Pocock N, Eisman J, Gwinn T et al (1989) Muscle strength, physical fitness, and weight but not age predict femoral neck bone mass. *Journal of Bone and Mineral Research* **4:** 441–448.

Ray WA, Griffin MR, Downey W & Melton LJ III (1989) Long-term use of thiazide diuretics and the risk of hip fracture. *Lancet* **i:** 687–690.

Riggs BL (1988) Osteoporosis. In Wyngaarden JB & Smith LH Jr (eds) *Cecil's Textbook of Medicine*, pp 1510–1515. Philadelphia: WB Saunders.

Riggs BL & Melton LJ III (1986) Medical progress: Involutional osteoporosis. *New England Journal of Medicine* **314:** 1676–1684.

Riggs BL & Melton LJ (1992) Involutional osteoporosis. In Evans JG & Williams TF (eds) *Oxford Textbook of Geriatric Medicine* (in press). Oxford: Oxford University Press.

Rigotti NA, Neer RM, Skates SJ, Herzog DB & Nussbaum SR (1991) The clinical course of osteoporosis in anorexia nervosa: A longitudinal study of cortical bone mass. *Journal of the American Medical Association* **265:** 1133–1138.

Ross PD, Wasnich RD & Vogel JM (1988) Detection of prefracture spinal osteoporosis using bone mineral absorptiometry. *Journal of Bone and Mineral Research* **3:** 1–11.

Ruff CB & Hayes WC (1982) Subperiosteal expansion and cortical remodeling of the human femur and tibia with aging. *Science* **217:** 945–948.

Seeley DG, Browner WS, Nevitt MC et al and the Study of Osteoporotic Fractures Research Group Universities of California (San Francisco), Pittsburgh, Maryland, Minnesota, and the Kaiser Permanente Center for Health Research, Portland, Oregon, USA (1990) In Christiansen C & Overgaard K (eds) *Osteoporosis 1990*, vol. 2, pp 463–464. Copenhagen: Osteopress ApS.

Seeman E, Melton LJ III, O'Fallon WM & Riggs BL (1983) Risk factors for spinal osteoporosis in men. *American Journal of Medicine* **75:** 977–983.

Seeman E, Cooper ME, Hopper JL et al (1988) Effect of early menopause on bone mass in normal women and patients with osteoporosis. *American Journal of Medicine* **85:** 213–216.

Simonen O (1988) Epidemiology and socio-economic aspects of osteoporosis in Finland. *Annales Chirurgiae et Gynaecologiae* **77:** 173–175.

Sinaki M (1988) Exercise and physical therapy. In Riggs BL & Melton LJ III (eds) *Osteoporosis: Etiology, Diagnosis, and Management*, pp 457–479. New York: Raven Press.

Slemenda CW, Hui SL, Longcope C, Wellman H & Johnston CC Jr (1990) Predictors of bone mass in perimenopausal women: A prospective study of clinical data using photon absorptiometry. *Annals of Internal Medicine* **112:** 96–101.

Solomon L (1979) Bone density in ageing Caucasian and African populations. *Lancet* **ii:** 1326–1330.

Sowers MF, Wallace RB & Lemke JH (1985a) Correlates of forearm bone mass among women during maximal bone mineralization. *Preventive Medicine* **14:** 585–596.

Sowers MF, Wallace RB & Lemke JH (1985b) Correlates of mid-radius bone density among postmenopausal women: A community study. *American Journal of Clinical Nutrition* **41:** 1045–1053.

Tinetti ME, Speechley M & Ginter SF (1988) Risk factors for falls among elderly persons living in the community. *New England Journal of Medicine* **319:** 1701–1707.

Turner RT, Greene VS & Bell NH (1987) Demonstration that ethanol inhibits bone matrix synthesis and mineralization in the rat. *Journal of Bone and Mineral Research* **2:** 61–66.

van Hemert AM, Vandenbroucke JP, Birkenhäger JC & Valkenburg HA (1990) Prediction of osteoporotic fractures in the general population by a fracture risk score: A 9-year follow-up among middle-aged women. *American Journal of Epidemiology* **132:** 123–135.

Wasnich RD, Benfante RJ, Yano K, Heilbrun L & Vogel JM (1983) Thiazide effect on the mineral content of bone. *New England Journal of Medicine* **309:** 344–347.

Wasnich RD, Ross PD, MacLean CJ, Davis JW & Vogel JM (1987) The relative strengths of osteoporotic risk factors in a prospective study of postmenopausal osteoporosis. In

Christiansen C, Johansen JS & Riis BJ (eds) *Osteoporosis 1987*, vol. 1, pp 394–395. Copenhagen: Osteopress ApS.

Yano K, Wasnich RD, Vogel JM & Heilbrun LK (1984) Bone mineral measurements among middle-aged and elderly Japanese residents in Hawaii. *American Journal of Epidemiology* **119**: 751–764.

2

Current techniques for bone mass measurement

CHRISTIAN HASSAGER
CLAUS CHRISTIANSEN

During the last three decades much effort has been spent on the development of methods for the quantitative assessment of the skeleton, which would enable early detection of osteoporosis, careful monitoring of its progression and response to therapy, and, perhaps most importantly, calculation of the present and future risk of fracture. Several methods are in current use; their precision and accuracy vary, and they measure bone with different ratios of trabecular and cortical bone. However, there is not yet a consensus on which method or methods are most efficacious for diagnosing and monitoring the individual patient or for screening large populations.

It is generally believed that the skeleton as a whole is composed of about 20% trabecular and 80% cortical bone. Trabecular bone has, compared with cortical bone, a high surface-to-volume ratio and therefore a presumed high turnover rate as well as a high responsiveness to metabolic and hormonal stimuli. The appendicular skeleton is mainly composed of cortical bone, although some areas, such as the distal radius end and the calcaneous have a high content of trabecular bone. In the spine trabecular bone predominates in the vertebral bodies, but the dense end plates and the posterior elements are mainly composed of cortical bone.

Epidemiological studies have shown that osteoporotic fractures occur first where trabecular bone predominates, such as in the vertebral body and the distal radius (Cummings et al, 1985; Riggs and Melton, 1989). This observation has led some authors to advocate that measurements for early detection of bone loss and for monitoring the response to therapy should be done at an anatomical site mainly composed of trabecular bone. However, definitive evidence for this statement is not available.

The first methods to be developed were radiogrammetry and single photon absorptiometry (SPA). These methods made it possible to measure the peripheral appendicular skeleton. In the past decade, techniques for the quantification of bone mineral content (BMC) anywhere in the skeleton have become available. Dual photon absorptiometry (DPA), and its off-spring dual energy X-ray absorptiometry (DEXA), can be used to measure the total cortical and trabecular BMC of any area of interest (typically the lumbar spine or the hip) or of the entire skeleton. The purely trabecular part of a bone (i.e. the vertebral spongiosum) can be measured by quantitative

Baillière's Clinical Obstetrics and Gynaecology—
Vol. 5, No. 4, December 1991
ISBN 0–7020–1548–2

Table 1. Comparison of techniques for bone mass measurement.

Technique	Site	Precision	Accuracy*
Single photon absorptiometry	Forearm/heel	1–2%	3–5%
Dual photon absorptiometry	AP spine/hip/total body	2–4%	5–10%
Dual energy X-ray absorptiometry	AP spine/lateral spine/hip/total body	1–3%	5–10%
Quantitative computed tomography	Spine (purely trabecular)	3–5%	5–20%

AP = anteroposterior.
* The accuracy values are estimated, as experimental data are sparse.

computed tomography (QCT). This chapter describes each of these methods, which are summarized in Table 1, and compares their utility for research as well as clinical use.

TECHNIQUES FOR BONE MASS MEASUREMENT

Radiogrammetry

The cortical thickness of a bone can be measured directly from a standard anteroposterior X-ray. This procedure (radiogrammetry), which is usually performed in the metacarpal shafts, is cheap, easy and reproducible (Meema, 1991). Cortical porosity and trabecular bone are, however, not measured by this technique, and changes in cortical thickness can only be accurately determined by this method in the appendicular skeleton.

Single photon absorptiometry

BMC measurements by single photon absorptiometry (SPA) depend on how much a photon beam is weakened by a bone. The most widely used energy source is iodine-125 (^{125}I), which has a photopeak at 27 KeV. SPA is primarily used for BMC determination in the forearm or the heel. SPA demands constant soft tissue thickness at the site of measurement. This may be solved by submerging the forearm or heel in water during the measurement, because lean soft tissue and water have similar absorption properties for ^{125}I photons. Both the attenuation coefficient and the density are, however, lower for fat than for lean soft tissue and water. Adequate fat correction, which can be done by a software routine (Hassager et al, 1989), is therefore essential if measurements are performed on obese subjects or on subjects that change their soft tissue body composition during the study period.

Most modern SPA devices use a ^{125}I source and a rectilinear scanning procedure. With this set-up the precision is 1–2%, depending on the measurement site (Figure 1). Measurements at the point where the radius–ulna gap is 8 mm and proximal thereto, where cortical bone predominates, can be done with a long-term precision of about 1% (Nilas et al, 1985). In the more trabecular areas, such as the heel and the ultradistal forearm, the

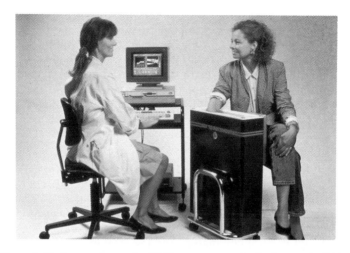

Figure 1. Modern equipment for BMC measurement in the forearm by SPA.

long-term precision is 1.5–2.0% (Nilas et al, 1985). The accuracy error of SPA measurements of excised bones is less than 2%.

Dual photon absorptiometry

The assumption of constant soft tissue thickness and composition, on which SPA is based, is not valid for measurements of the axial skeleton. Dual photon absorptiometry (DPA), which uses two distinct photon energies instead of one, can partially solve this problem. However, one assumption is still needed. The pixels next to the bones are used for baseline determination. The composition (fat/lean ratio) of the soft tissue in these pixels is then assumed to be equal to the composition of the soft tissue in the pixels that contain bone.

A rectilinear scan pattern is also used for DPA measurements. The subject lies on a scan table with a radiation source moving under the table and a detector moving above. Gadolinium-153 (^{153}Gd), with principal photopeaks at 44 KeV and 100 KeV, is the most commonly used radiation source. The typical scanning time is 30–45 min.

DPA measurements can theoretically be performed on any area of interest of the body. The most commonly used areas are the lumbar (L_2–L_4) spine and various areas of the hip (trochanter, femoral neck and Ward's triangle). The measured values are given as BMC (in grams) or as bone mineral density (BMD), which is BMC divided by the projected area of the bone (in g/cm^2). BMD is thus not a true density, but merely a BMC corrected for the number of pixels in which it is measured.

The long-term in vivo precision is 3–4% with rigid quality assurance (Nilas et al, 1988), but problems related to source changes may increase the precision error even further. With an average source life of only 1 year, this is a real problem. Several studies (Dunn et al, 1980; Wahner et al, 1985;

Gotfredsen et al, 1988) have shown a good in vitro accuracy (3–5%) for DPA, but only one study has examined the more relevant in situ accuracy (Gotfredsen et al, 1988). From measurements on 13 whole cadavers the accuracy of BMC and BMD measured by DPA was found to be 8–10%. The relative higher in situ accuracy error can be caused by several factors. First, the assumption of similar soft tissue body composition in the bone and non-bone pixels may not be completely valid. Furthermore, DPA measurements may be affected by aortic calcification and osteophytes.

Dual energy X-ray absorptiometry

Dual energy X-ray absorptiometry (DEXA) is now replacing DPA at most institutions. DEXA is based on the same principle as DPA, but used an X-ray tube instead of an isotope as the photon source. Because of the increased photon flux from an X-ray tube compared with an isotope source, the scanning time is decreased to 4–5 min for a spine or hip measurement, the X-ray beam is more collimated, and the scan image sharper. This has resulted in improved precision compared with DPA. The precision is about 1.0–1.5% for an anteroposterior projection of the spine (Hansen et al, 1990; Orwoll et al, 1991) and 1–3% for the hip (Orwoll et al, 1991).

Direct in situ accuracy studies have not yet been performed for DEXA. The in vitro accuracy error of DEXA measurements on excised vertebral bodies was recently found to be about 9% (Ho et al, 1990). Inhomogeneous soft tissue body composition, aortic calcification and osteophytes, which result in inaccuracy in DPA measurements, will of course also affect the accuracy of DEXA measurements.

The increased photon flux has also made measurement of the lateral projection of the spine more accessible. The advantage of a 'lateral spine' measurement is that it is possible to perform isolated measurements on the vertebral body without inclusion of the posterior spinal elements. However, in most patients only one or two vertebral bodies project free of the ribs and the pelvis. The precision error of a lateral spine measurement by DEXA is about 3% (Slosman et al, 1990), and the accuracy is unknown. An accurate lateral measurement may be more difficult to perform because of the increased ratio of soft tissue to bone for this projection compared with a traditional anteroposterior projection.

Quantitative computed tomography

Quantitative computed tomography (QCT) measurements of bone mineral are performed on standard computed tomography (CT) scanners, but sophisticated calibration and positioning are required in order to get quantitative information from the CT image. QCT has the ability to distinguish cortical and trabecular bone. A typical spine measurement, where a few cubic centimetres of purely trabecular bone in two to four vertebral bodies $(T_{12}-L_4)$ are quantified and averaged, takes about 10 min. A calibration phantom is measured simultaneously with the patient to correct for scanner instability. QCT has also been used for hip measurements, but this application has only been scarcely investigated.

Both single and dual energy QCT are available. The in vivo precision is 2–3% for single energy QCT and at least 3–5% for dual energy QCT (Genant et al, 1982). The in vitro accuracy of single energy QCT ranges from 5 to 15% in human vertebral specimens, but the accuracy error in vivo in elderly osteoporotic patients may be as high as 20 to 30%. A major source of inaccuracy is the variable amount of fat in the marrow. Dual energy QCT can reduce the magnitude of this error, but at the expense of reduced precision (Genant and Boyd, 1977).

The radiation dose received from one single energy QCT measurement is much higher (about 200 mrem) than that received from one SPA, DPA or DEXA measurement (10 mrem or less). This feature may limit the use of QCT for repeated measurements in longitudinal studies.

COMPARISON OF THE UTILITY OF THE TECHNIQUES

The purpose of bone mass measurements may be either to *diagnose* low bone mass in order to predict present or future fracture risk, or to *follow up* changes in bone mass to determine spontaneous bone loss or to monitor the effect of a treatment. When evaluating a technique for follow-up purposes the most important parameter is the precision or reproducibility of the method. It can be calculated that the minimum detectable significant difference (5% level) between two measurements in a single subject is 2.8% if the precision error is 1%, and 14% if the precision error is 5% (Figure 2a). A bone loss of 3% per year, which is the average normal bone loss in the early postmenopause, would therefore take 1 year to detect with a 1% precision error and 4.7 years with a 5% precision error if only two measurements are made. Groups of patients are often studied for research purpose. When the biological variation in the change in bone mass is ignored,

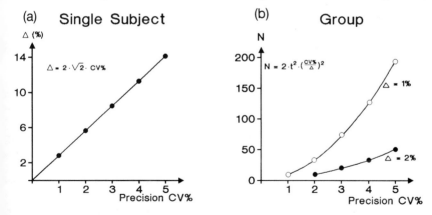

Figure 2. (a) The relationship between the precision error of the method (precision CV) and the minimal detectable (5% significance level) difference ($\triangle$) between two measurements in one subject. (b) The relationship between the precision error of the method (precision CV) and the number of subjects (N) in a group needed to detect (5% significance level) a change of 1% or 2%.

detection on a group basis of an 1% difference between two measurements in each subject would demand approximately 10 subjects with a 1% precision error, and 200 subjects with a 5% precision error (Figure 2b). Although the biological variation would increase both these numbers, the lower one (10) relatively more than the higher one (200), this example clearly shows that high precision methodology can mean a saving in research resources.

In some cases there may be a special interest in a certain region of the skeleton and theoretically the most optimal way of studying this is to determine the BMC in that particular region. The calculations above demonstrate, however, that this may not always be the case. It may be better to measure the BMC in another region if this can be done with more precision than BMC measurements in the region of interest. It depends on the correlation between the changes in the two regions as well as the difference in the ratio of the change to the precision of the two methods. DEXA has now reduced the precision error of a spinal BMC measurement to about 1%, i.e. the same range as appendicular SPA measurements. Direct spinal DEXA measurements may therefore be preferred to appendicular SPA measurements, if the only aim is to study changes in spinal BMC. Serial appendicular SPA measurements may, however, reflect changes in total skeletal mass just as well as serial local DEXA measurements.

Bone mass measurements may also be used for diagnostic purposes, i.e. to predict present and future fracture risk, but for this the measured values must be interpreted with care. As mentioned elsewhere in this issue, postmenopausal osteoporosis is a major health hazard in elderly women that may be prevented by oestrogen substitution therapy, but effective treatment of developed disease does not yet exist. There are, however, still doubts about the possible risks of long-term oestrogen replacement therapy (Barrett-Connor, 1989). Appropriate screening tests before bone loss occurs, i.e. at the time of the menopause, to identify the women most likely to suffer a future fracture are therefore needed.

There are probably two major determinants of fracture risk which relate to the bone mass: the peak adult bone mass and the postmenopausal rate of bone loss. The relationship between peak adult bone mass and the risk of future fractures has still to be established, although several prospective studies have shown that low bone mass in elderly women increases the risk of fragility fractures (Hui et al, 1988; Ross et al, 1988; Cummings et al, 1990). The rate of bone loss can be determined by repeated measurements of bone mass, and in perimenopausal women it may be estimated by biochemical indices of bone turnover (Christiansen et al, 1987), but its relationship to subsequent fractures is unknown.

There are only a few prospective studies that have evaluated the relationship between bone mass and fracture risk (Hui et al, 1988; Ross et al, 1988; Cummings et al, 1990). These studies have not demonstrated superiority of one type of bone mass measurement over another in the prediction of whether a subject will suffer a fracture or not in the near future.

A more indirect way of studying the diagnostic value of a bone mass measurement is to compare values in age-matched fracture and non-fracture cases. All known methods for bone mass measurements show a large overlap between the measured values in these two groups. These type of studies have resulted in considerable disagreement as to which part of the skeleton should be measured in order to determine the risk of future fracture. The forearm is simpler and less expensive to measure than the spine, but as spinal compression fracture is one of the commonest osteoporotic fractures, many advocate spinal measurements, and some studies (Riggs et al, 1981; Eastell et al, 1989) have found better discrimination of fracture and non-fracture cases with the use of spinal instead of appendicular measurements. A number of other studies (Ott et al, 1987; Nordin et al, 1988; Gotfredsen et al, 1989) have, however, shown that, whereas appendicular bone mass measurements only correlate moderately well with those of the spine, they are equally able to separate non-fractured and fractured cases—even fractures in the spine. The results from one such study are given in Figure 3, where it can be seen that forearm SPA measurements separate fracture and non-fracture cases as well as spinal DEXA measurements do. QCT measurement of purely trabecular bone in the spine has been reported to separate patients with mild and defined vertebral fracture cases slightly better than spinal SPA measurements and forearm SPA measurements do (Heuck et al, 1989). Longitudinal data are, however, lacking for this technique, and the most recent osteoporosis consensus report (Consensus Development Conference, 1990) states: 'It is now established that a single accurate measurement of bone mass at any site has equal predictive value for subsequent fractures of all types.'

The diagnosis of osteoporosis affecting a specific site of the skeleton may require bone mass measurement at that site. For example, if vertebral

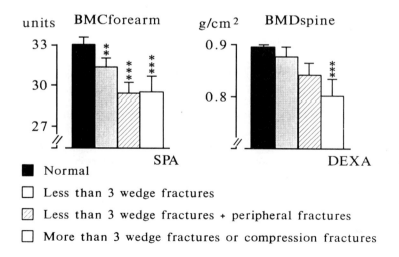

Figure 3. Bone mineral content of the forearm (BMC forearm) and bone mineral density of the lumbar spine (BMD spine) in 387 elderly postmenopausal women. Difference from normal: $** = P < 0.01$; $*** = P < 0.001$. From Overgaard et al (1992), with permission.

deformities are detected on a radiograph, measurement of spinal bone mass may be necessary to determine whether significant spinal osteoporosis is present. This is based on the not very powerful (i.e. $r = 0.5$–0.7) correlation between measured spinal bone mass and measured appendicular bone mass. The accuracy error of in vivo spinal measurements is, however, not clearly determined yet, and some data indicate that for DPA measurements it may be as high as 8–10% (Gotfredsen et al, 1988). Correlation between measured spinal bone mass and appendicular bone mass therefore cannot be expected to be perfect, and part of the error in the prediction of spinal bone mass from an appendicular bone mass measurement may thus be caused by inaccuracy of the spinal measurement itself.

REFERENCES

Barrett-Connor E (1989) Postmenopausal estrogen replacement and breast cancer. *New England Journal of Medicine* **321:** 319–320.

Christiansen C, Riis BJ & Rødbro P (1987) Prediction of rapid bone loss in postmenopausal women. *Lancet* **i:** 1105–1108.

Consensus Development Conference (1991) Prophylaxis and treatment of osteoporosis. *American Journal of Medicine* **90:** 107–110.

Cummings SR, Kelsey JL, Nevitt MC & O'Dowd KJ (1985) Epidemiology of osteoporosis and osteoporotic fractures. *Epidemiologic Reviews* **7:** 178–208.

Cummings SR, Black DM, Nevitt MC et al (1990) Appendicular bone density and age predict hip fracture in women. *Journal of the American Medical Association* **263:** 665–668.

Dunn WL, Wahner HW & Riggs BL (1980) Measurement of bone mineral content in human vertebrae and hip by dual photon absorptiometry. *Radiology* **136:** 485–487.

Eastell R, Wahner HW, O'Fallon M, Amadio PC, Melton LJ III & Riggs BL (1989) Unequal decrease in bone density of lumbar spine and ultradistal radius in Colles' and vertebral fracture syndromes. *Journal of Clinical Investigation* **83:** 168–174.

Genant HK & Boyd DP (1977) Quantitative bone mineral analysis using dual-energy computed tomography. *Investigative Radiology* **12:** 545.

Genant HK, Cann CE, Ettinger B & Gordan GS (1982) Quantitative computed tomography of vertebral spongiosa: A sensitive method for detecting early bone loss after oophorectomy. *Annals of Internal Medicine* **97:** 699–705.

Gotfredsen A, Pødenphant J, Nørgaard H, Nilas L, Nielsen VH & Christiansen C (1988) Accuracy of lumbar spine bone mineral content by dual photon absorptiometry. *Journal of Nuclear Medicine* **29:** 248–254.

Gotfredsen A, Pødenphant J, Nilas L & Christiansen C (1989) Discriminative ability of total body bone-mineral measured by dual photon absorptiometry. *Scandinavian Journal of Clinical and Laboratory Investigation* **49:** 125–134.

Hansen MA, Hassager C, Overgaard K, Marslew U, Riis BJ & Christiansen C (1990) Dual-energy x-ray absorptiometry: A precise method of measuring bone mineral density in the lumbar spine. *Journal of Nuclear Medicine* **31:** 1156–1162.

Hassager C, Borg J & Christiansen C (1989) Measurement of the subcutaneous fat in the distal forearm by single photon absorptiometry. *Metabolism: Clinical and Experimental* **38:** 159–165.

Heuck A, Block M, Glüer CC et al (1989) Mild versus definite osteoporosis: Comparison of bone densitometry techniques using different statistical models. *Journal of Bone and Mineral Research* **4:** 891–900.

Ho CP, Kim RW, Schaffer MB & Sartoris DJ (1990) Accuracy of dual-energy radiographic absorptiometry of the lumbar spine: Cadaver study. *Radiology* **176:** 171–173.

Hui SL, Slemenda CW & Johnson CC Jr (1988) Age and bone mass as predictors of fracture in a prospective study. *Journal of Clinical Investigation* **81:** 1804–1809.

Meema HE (1991) Improved vertebral fracture threshold in postmenopausal osteoporosis by radiogrammetric measurements: Its usefulness in selection for preventive therapy. *Journal of Bone and Mineral Research* **6:** 9–14.

Nilas L, Borg J, Gotfredsen A & Christiansen C (1985) Comparison of single- and dual-photon absorptiometry in postmenopausal bone mineral loss. *Journal of Nuclear Medicine* **26:** 1257–1262.

Nilas L, Hassager C & Christiansen C (1988) Long-term precision of dual photon absorptiometry in the lumbar spine in clinical settings. *Bone and Mineral* **3:** 305–315.

Nordin BEC, Wishart JM, Horowith M, Need AG, Bridges A & Bellon M (1988) The relation between forearm and vertebral mineral density and fractures in postmenopausal women. *Bone and Mineral* **5:** 21–33.

Orwoll ES, Oviatt SK & the Nafarelin/Bone Study Group (1991) Longitudinal precision of dual-energy x-ray absorptiometry in a multicenter study. *Journal of Bone and Mineral Research* **6:** 191–197.

Ott SM, Kilcoyne RF & Chesnut CH (1987) Ability of four different techniques of measuring bone mass to diagnose vertebral fractures in postmenopausal women. *Journal of Bone and Mineral Research* **2:** 201–210.

Overgaard K, Hansen MA, Riis BJ & Christiansen C (1992) Discriminatory ability of bone mass measurements (SPA and DEXA) for fractures in elderly postmenopausal women. *Calcified Tissue International* **50:** 30–35.

Riggs BL & Melton LJ III (1986) Medical progress: Involutional osteoporosis. *New England Journal of Medicine* **314:** 1676–1686.

Riggs BL, Wahner HW, Dunn WL, Mazess RB, Offord KP & Melton LJ (1981) Differential changes in bone mineral density of the appendicular and axial skeleton with aging. *Journal of Clinical Investigation* **67:** 328–335.

Ross PD, Wasnish RD & Vogel JM (1988) Detection of prefracture spinal osteoporosis using bone mineral absorptiometry. *Journal of Bone and Mineral Research* **3:** 1–11.

Slosman DO, Rizzoli R, Donath A & Bonjour J-Ph (1990) Vertebral bone mineral density measured laterally by dual-energy x-ray absorptiometry. *Osteoporosis International* **1:** 23–29.

Wahner HW, Dunn WL, Mazess RB et al (1985) Dual photon Gd-153 absorptiometry of bone. *Radiology* **156:** 203–206.

3

What do we know about biochemical bone markers?

P. D. DELMAS

Bone metabolism is characterized by two opposite activities: the formation of new bone by osteoblasts, and the degradation (resorption) of old bone by osteoclasts. Both are tightly coupled in time and space in a sequence of events which define the remodelling unit. Bone mass depends on the balance between resorption and formation within a remodelling unit and on the number of remodelling units which are activated within a given period of time in a defined area of bone. Needless to say, bone formation and bone resorption are altered in most metabolic bone diseases, including osteoporosis.

Invasive techniques measuring bone turnover have provided useful information, but all of them have limitations. Histomorphometry of the iliac crest provides unique information on the rate of formation at the cellular and tissue level, and allows measurement of the frequency of activation of remodelling units, but the assessment of bone resorption is less accurate. In addition, measurement of bone turnover is limited to a small area of the cancellous bone and the corticoendosteal envelope, which may not reflect bone turnover in other parts of the skeleton (Delmas, 1988). Calcium kinetic studies have allowed the quantification of the increase in bone turnover after the menopause, but measurement of the calcium accretion rate—an index of bone formation—may be inaccurate in elderly women (Eastell et al, 1988). Finally, the whole body retention of labelled bisphosphonates, a marker of bone turnover and bone formation has not proved to be very sensitive (Thomsen et al, 1987). These limitations, in addition to the need for non-invasive techniques that can be applied more widely and repeated several times in a single patient, explain the development of markers of bone turnover which can be measured in blood and urine.

In contrast to metabolic bone diseases such as Paget's disease of bone or renal osteodystrophy which are characterized by dramatic changes in bone turnover, in osteoporosis subtle modifications of the bone remodelling activity can lead to a substantial loss of bone mass after a long period of time. This explains why most conventional markers are normal, for example, in a woman with a well-characterized vertebral osteoporosis who has recently undergone the menopause. Consequently there have been efforts to develop more sensitive biochemical markers of bone turnover.

Baillière's Clinical Obstetrics and Gynaecology—
Vol. 5, No. 4, December 1991
ISBN 0–7020–1548–2

The rate of formation or degradation of the bone matrix can be assessed either by measuring a prominent enzymatic activity of the bone-forming or resorbing cells—such as alkaline and acid phosphatase activity—or by measuring bone matrix components released into the circulation during formation or resorption (Table 1). As discussed below, these markers are of varying specificity and sensitivity, and some of them have not yet been fully investigated. In addition, because circulating levels of these markers can be influenced by factors other than bone turnover, such as their metabolic clearance, their clinical significance should be validated by comparison with direct assessment of bone formation and resorption by iliac crest histo-morphometry and/or calcium kinetic studies, keeping in mind the limitations of these techniques. Finally, the possibility of combining these new markers of bone turnover with the measurement of bone mass by absorptiometry (see Chapter 2) offers an exciting opportunity to assess more efficiently the risk of osteoporosis in women at the time of menopause and to monitor the effect of hormone replacement therapy (HRT).

Table 1. Biochemical markers of bone turnover.

Formation	Resorption
Most efficient markers:	*Most efficient markers*:
Serum osteocalcin (bone gla-protein)	Urinary pyridinoline and deoxypyridinoline
Total and bone-specific alkaline phos-phatase	(collagen crosslinks)
	Total and dialysable urinary hydroxyproline
Other markers:	*Other markers*:
Serum procollagen I extension peptides (carboxyterminal)	Plasma tartrate-resistant acid phosphatase
Other non-collagenous bone proteins (?)	Urinary hydroxylysine glycosides
	Free γ-carboxyglutamic acid
	Fragments of non-collagenous proteins (?)

BIOCHEMICAL MARKERS OF BONE FORMATION

Serum alkaline phosphatase

Serum alkaline phosphatase activity is the most commonly used marker of bone formation, but it lacks sensitivity and specificity, especially in patients with osteoporosis (Table 1). Also, a moderate increase in serum alkaline phosphatase is ambiguous as it may reflect a mineralization defect in elderly patients, or may be the result of one of the numerous medications which have been shown to increase the hepatic isoenzyme of alkaline phosphatase. In an attempt to improve the specificity and the sensitivity of serum alkaline phosphatase measurement, techniques have been developed to differentiate the bone and liver isoenzymes, which differ only in post-translational modifications as they are coded by a single gene. These techniques rely on the use of differentially effective activators and inhibitors (heat, phenyl-alaline and urea), separation by electrophoresis and separation by specific antibodies (Farley et al, 1981; Moss, 1982; Duda et al, 1988). In general, these assays have slightly enhanced the sensitivity of this marker, but most of them are indirect and/or technically cumbersome. A real improvement should be obtained by using a monoclonal antibody which recognizes the bone but not the liver and kidney isoenzyme, a reagent which has recently become available (Hill and Wolfert, 1989).

Serum osteocalcin

Osteocalcin, also called bone gla-protein (BGP), is a small, non-collagenous protein which is specific for bone tissue and dentine, but its precise function remains unknown (Price, 1987). Osteocalcin is predominately synthesized by osteoblasts and is incorporated into the extracellular matrix of bone, but a fraction of neosynthesized osteocalcin is released into the circulation, where it can be measured by radioimmunoassay (Price et al, 1980; Delmas et al, 1983; Lian and Gundberg, 1988). Because antibodies directed against bovine osteocalcin cross react with human osteocalcin, most systems have been developed with bovine osteocalcin as a tracer, standard and immunogen. Depending on the epitopes recognized by the antibody, some polyclonal antisera, and also some monoclonal antibodies may detect fragments of osteocalcin in addition to the intact molecule. Some of these fragments may be released during bone resorption in a high turnover state (Gundberg and Weinstein, 1986), but some of them are unrelated to resorption and are of unknown significance (Tracy et al, 1990). In our experience, most polyclonal antibodies raised against the intact molecule do not recognize significant amounts of osteocalcin fragments in serum from patients with osteoporosis and other bone diseases, with the exception of chronic renal failure. This pattern implies that such an assay is a valid marker of bone turnover when resorption and formation are coupled, and that it is a specific marker of bone formation whenever formation and resorption are uncoupled, such as in multiple myeloma and in some patients with vertebral osteoporosis (Brown et al, 1984; Delmas et al, 1985, 1986; Bataille et al, 1987). Several investigators, including ourselves, have found that serum osteocalcin is significantly higher during the night than during the day. Using our antiserum R102, we have found that serum osteocalcin undergoes a circadian rhythm within a narrow range, with a nightly peak at 4 a.m., a nadir at 5 p.m. and a 15% difference between peak and trough (Delmas et al, 1987). This circadian rhythm is likely to reflect an increase in bone turnover during the night, as shown previously with other markers of bone turnover. Interestingly, a significant effect of the menstrual cycle has been recently reported (Nielsen et al, 1990), with an increase in serum osteocalcin during the luteal period. Finally, it has been suggested that urinary osteocalcin determination might be valuable in some clinical situations (Taylor et al, 1990).

Procollagen I extension peptides

During the extracellular processing of collagen I, there is cleavage of the aminoterminal (p coll-I-N) and carboxyterminal (p coll-I-C) extension peptides prior to fibril formation. These peptides circulate in blood, where they might represent useful markers of bone formation, as collagen is by far the most abundant organic component of bone matrix. Using a radio-immunoassay for p coll-I-C, it has been shown that a single dose of 30 mg of prednisone suppresses serum p coll-I-C without decreasing urinary hydroxyproline (Simon and Krane, 1983). This suggests that circulating p coll-I-C levels do indeed reflect bone formation. Serum p coll-I-C is weakly correlated with histological bone formation, with r values ranging from 0.36 to 0.50 in patients with vertebral osteoporosis (Parfitt et al, 1987). The effect of menopause on serum p coll-I-C is not clearly documented, and currently available assays may not be sensitive enough for the investigation of osteoporosis.

An assay for p coll-I-N using a synthetic peptide as an immunogen has been recently reported, but data in osteoporosis are not yet available (Kraenzlin et al, 1989). It should be noted that, in contrast to what was initially believed, a fraction of p coll-I-N is incorporated into the bone matrix, where it has been identified as the 24 kDa phosphoprotein of bone. Therefore, the release of fragments of p coll-I-N during resorption might be a source of serum immunoreactivity of p coll-I-N according to the epitope seen by a given antiserum. In addition, the clearance and metabolism of these peptides is unknown. Further studies are necessary to assess the potential use of procollagen I extension peptides in detecting the increase of bone turnover at the menopause and the abnormalities of bone formation in patients with osteoporosis.

Other bone proteins

Osteonectin and bone sialoprotein II (BSP) are two major bone-related proteins secreted by osteoblasts, and are potential markers of bone for-mation. They circulate in blood, where they can be measured by radio-immunoassay (Stenner et al, 1986; Malaval et al, 1987; Chenu and Delmas, 1990). Unfortunately, platelets contain significant amounts of osteonectin and BSP, which make a major contribution to the levels detected in serum (Stenner et al, 1986; Chenu and Delmas, 1990). Monoclonal antibodies capable of recognizing osteonectin and BSP from bone but not from platelet origin might be useful and need to be evaluated (Malaval et al, 1988).

BIOCHEMICAL MARKERS OF BONE RESORPTION

Urinary hydroxyproline

Hydroxyproline is found mainly in collagens and represents about 13% of the amino acid content of the molecule (Prockop and Kivirikko, 1968). Hydroxyproline is derived from proline by a post-translational hydroxyl-ation occurring within the peptide chain. Because free hydroxyproline released during the degradation of collagen cannot be reutilized in collagen synthesis, most of the endogenous hydroxyproline present in biological fluids is derived from the degradation of various forms of collagen (Prockop et al, 1979). As half of human collagen resides in bone, where its turnover is probably faster than in soft tissues, excretion of hydroxyproline in urine is regarded as a marker of bone resorption. Actually, the C1q fraction of complement contains significant amounts of hydroxyproline and could account for up to 40% of urinary hydroxyproline. The relationship of urinary hydroxyproline to the metabolism of collagen is more complex. Hydroxyproline is present in biological fluids in different forms. About 90% of the hydroxyproline released by the breakdown of collagen in the tissues, and especially during bone resorption, is degraded to the free amino acid that circulates in plasma, is filtered, and is almost entirely reabsorbed by the kidney. It is eventually completely oxidized in the liver and is degraded to carbon dioxide and urea (Kivirikko, 1983; Lowry et al, 1985). About 10% of the hydroxyproline released by the breakdown of collagen circulates in the peptide-bound form, and these hydroxyproline-containing peptides are filtered and excreted in urine without any further metabolism. Thus, the urinary total hydroxyproline represents only about 10% of total collagen catabolism. Hydroxyproline is present in urine in three forms: free hydroxy-proline, small hydroxyproline-containing peptides that are dialysable and represent over 90% of the total urinary excretion of this amino acid, and a small number of non-dialysable polypeptides containing hydroxyproline (Prockop and Kivirikko, 1968). Colorimetric assay of hydroxyproline is usually performed on a hydrolysed urine sample and therefore reflects the total excretion of the amino acid. As a consequence of its tissue origin and metabolism pattern, urinary hydroxyproline is poorly correlated with bone resorption as assessed by calcium kinetics or bone histomorphometry (Delmas, 1990) and there is an obvious need for a more sensitive marker of bone resorption.

Urinary hydroxylysine glycosides

Hydroxylysine is another amino acid unique to collagen and proteins containing collagen-like sequences. Like hydroxyproline, hydroxylysine is not reutilized for collagen biosynthesis and, although it is much less abundant than hydroxyproline, it is a potential marker of collagen degradation. Hydroxylysine is present in part as galactosyl hydroxylysine and in part as glucosyl-galactosyl hydroxylysine. The relative proportions and total content of galactosyl hydroxylysine and glucosyl-galactosyl hydroxylysine varies in bone and soft tissues, which suggests that their urinary excretion might be a more sensitive marker of bone resorption than urinary hydroxy-proline. Urinary galactosyl hydroxylysine increases with ageing (Moro et al, 1988a) and might be a useful marker in patients with osteoporosis (Moro et al, 1988b). This marker deserves further evaluation in osteoporosis.

Plasma tartrate-resistant acid phosphatase

Acid phosphatase is a lysosomal enzyme that is present primarily in bone, prostate, platelets, erythrocytes and the spleen. These different isoenzymes can be separated by electrophoretic methods, but these lack sensitivity and specificity. The bone acid phosphatase is resistant to L(+)-tartrate, whereas the prostatic isoenzyme is inhibited (Li et al, 1973). Acid phosphatase circulates in blood and shows a higher activity in serum than in plasma because of the release of platelet phosphatase activity during the clotting process. In normal plasma, tartrate-resistant acid phosphatase (TRAP) corresponds to plasma isoenzyme 5, which originates partly from bone. Osteoclasts contain a tartrate-resistant acid phosphatase that is released into the circulation (Minkin, 1982). Plasma TRAP is increased in a variety of metabolic bone disorders with increased bone turnover (Stepan et al, 1983), and is elevated after oophorectomy (Stepan et al, 1987) and in vertebral osteoporosis (Piedra et al, 1989), but it is not clear whether this marker is actually more sensitive than urinary hydroxyproline (Stepan et al, 1987). Its clinical utility in osteoporosis remains to be investigated. The lack of specificity of plasma TRAP activity for the osteoclast, its instability in frozen samples and the presence of enzyme inhibitors in serum are potential drawbacks which will limit the development of enzymatic assays of TRAP. Conversely, the development of new immunoassays using monoclonal antibodies specifically directed against the bone isoenzyme of TRAP (Kraenzlin, 1990) should be valuable in assessing the ability of this marker to predict osteoclast activity in osteoporosis.

Serum γ-carboxyglutamic acid

γ-Carboxyglutamic acid (gla) results from the vitamin K-dependent post-translational modification of some glutamic acid residues in at least two bone proteins (osteocalcin and matrix gla-protein), in some coagulation factors (factors II, VII, IX and X) and in plasma proteins C, S and Z. Increased levels of urinary gla have been reported in patients with osteoporosis, but its significance has not been fully investigated (Gundberg et al, 1983). Using an original assay involving O-phthalaldehyde derivatization of plasma, reversed-phase high pressure liquid chromatography (HPLC) and detection of the gla peak by fluorimetry, we have shown that free gla circulates in blood with a mean level in adults of 167 ± 46 pmol/ml (Fournier et al, 1989). Free gla in the serum is increased in patients with primary hyperpara-thyroidism and Paget's disease of bone. Free gla in the serum originates both from the metabolism of the vitamin K-dependent clotting factors and from bone metabolism (Fournier et al, 1989), and the fraction derived from bone is related to bone resorption and not to formation (unpublished data). However, because of its mixed origin, serum levels of free gla are not sensitive enough to assess the subtle changes in bone resorption which occur in osteoporosis.

Urinary excretion of the collagen pyridinium crosslink

Pyridinoline (Pyr) and deoxypyridinoline (D-Pyr), also called respectively hydroxylysylpyridinoline (HP) and lysylpyridinoline (LP), are the two irreducible pyridinium crosslinks present in the mature form of collagen (Eyre, 1987). This post-translational covalent cross-linking generated from lysine and hydroxylysine residues is unique to collagen and elastin molecules. It creates interchain bonds which stabilize the molecule. The concentration of Pyr and D-Pyr in connective tissues is very low and varies dramatically with tissue type. Pyr is widely distributed in the type I collagen of bone and in the type II collagen of cartilage, and is found in smaller amounts in other connective tissues, except skin. Most interestingly, D-Pyr has only been found in significant amounts in the type I collagen of bone, at a concentration of 0.07 mol/mol of collagen (Eyre et al, 1984, 1988). Pyr and D-Pyr are excreted in urine in peptide-bound and free forms and their total amounts can be measured by fluorimetry after reversed-phase HPLC of a cellulose-bound extract of hydrolysed urine (Eyre et al, 1984; Black et al, 1988). With such an assay, we have shown that urinary Pyr and D-Pyr represent a more sensitive marker of bone resorption than hydroxyproline in Paget's disease of bone and primary hyperparathyroidism (Uebelhart et al, 1990). When compared with urinary hydroxyproline, the measurement of urinary Pyr and D-Pyr has several potential advantages: their relative specificity for bone turnover and the fact that they do not appear to be metabolized in vivo prior to their urinary excretion should allow a precise assessment of the amount of bone which is resorbed. Also, the absence of intestinal absorption of Pyr and D-Pyr contained in gelatine allows the measurement of levels in urine without any food restriction (Colwell et al, 1990). As discussed below, urinary Pyr and D-Pyr are promising markers for the assessment of bone resorption in osteoporosis and at the menopause. More information is needed about their clearance, especially when the glomerular filtration rate is decreased, a common finding in the elderly. A more convenient assay is mandatory if this measurement is to be developed on a large scale.

CHANGES IN BONE TURNOVER AT THE MENOPAUSE

Bone turnover increases in normal women from the fourth to the tenth decade, as shown by the gradual increase in serum total and bone-specific alkaline phosphatase, osteocalcin and urinary hydroxyproline (Delmas et al, 1983). This pattern has also been documented by the increase in bone formation and resorption measured on iliac crest biopsy in normal women in their late sixties compared with women in their thirties (Eastell et al, 1988). Superimposed on the effect of ageing, the menopause induces a dramatic increase in bone turnover which peaks 1 to 3 years after cessation of ovarian function and slows down thereafter for the next 8–10 years, a pattern which is also illustrated by cross-sectional studies after oophorectomy (Stepan et al, 1987). Serum osteocalcin, urinary pyridinoline crosslinks and other markers of bone turnover are significantly increased after the menopause and return to premenopausal levels within a few months of HRT (Johansen et al, 1988; Uebelhart et al, 1991) (Figures 1 and 2). Two independent studies have shown that in untreated postmenopausal women followed for 2 to 4 years, serum osteocalcin is the best single biochemical marker reflecting the spontaneous rate of bone loss as assessed by repeated measurements of the bone mineral content of the radius and the lumbar spine, i.e. the higher

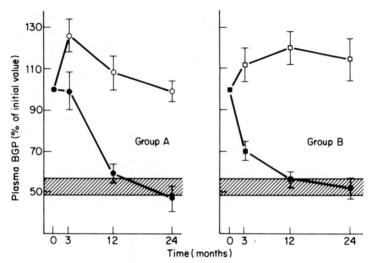

Figure 1. Plasma BGP levels in 110 healthy early postmenopausal women as a function of time in two treatment groups. The closed circles represent percutaneous 17β-oestradiol (group A), and the closed boxes represent oral 17β-oestradiol (group B); the open symbols represent placebo treatment. For each subject the initial plasma BGP value concentration was set at 100% and all subsequent values were expressed as a percentage of each initial value. Bars are ±1 SEM. The hatched areas indicate the mean (±1 SEM) BGP values obtained from 39 healthy and age-matched (45–54 years) premenopausal women expressed as a percentage of the initial mean values of the postmenopausal women. From Johansen et al (1988), with permission.

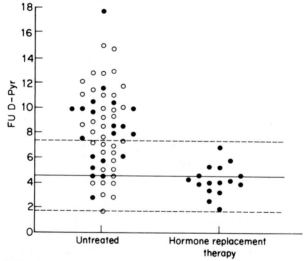

Figure 2. Individual values of fasting urinary (FU) D-Pyr (in pmol/μmol creatinine) in 57 untreated postmenopausal women are shown on the left. Values for 16 women before (left) and after (right) 6 months of hormone replacement therapy are represented by the black circles. The horizontal lines represent the range of fasting D-Pyr of age-matched premenopausal women (mean value given as a solid line and ±2SD as dashed lines). From Uebelhart et al (1991), with permission.

the bone turnover rate, the higher the rate of bone loss (Slemenda et al, 1987; Johansen et al, 1988). Recently, we have shown that the combination of a single measurement of serum osteocalcin, urinary hydroxyproline and urinary D-Pyr can predict the rate of bone loss over 2 years with an r value of 0.77 (Uebelhart et al, 1991) (Figure 3). Whether slow and fast losers of bone do so for a prolonged period of time after the menopause is debated and should be assessed by more long-term, prospective studies. The combination of bone mass measurement and the assessment of bone turnover by a battery of specific markers is likely to be helpful in the future for the screening of patients at risk for osteoporosis to detect those who should be treated.

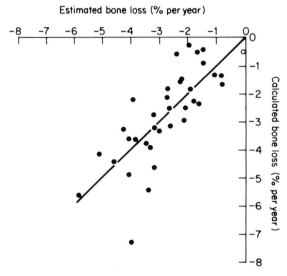

Figure 3. Correlation between the calculated rate of bone loss (percent per year) and the estimated rate of bone loss using the initial fasting D-Pyr, hydroxyproline and plasma osteocalcin measurements in 36 early postmenopausal women. The calculated rate of bone loss was obtained by repeated measurement of bone mineral density of the forearm over 2 years in women who did not receive any specific treatment such as hormone replacement therapy. $r = 0.77$; $n = 36$. From Uebelhart et al (1991), with permission.

BONE TURNOVER IN POSTMENOPAUSAL WOMEN WITH VERTEBRAL OSTEOPOROSIS

In patients with untreated vertebral osteoporosis, there is a wide scatter beyond the normal range of individual values of biochemical markers of bone turnover which reflects the histological heterogeneity of the disease. Serum osteocalcin is in the lower range of normal in patients with a low osteoblastic activity and significantly increased in the one-third of patients who have a high bone turnover. When serum BGP is compared with the bone remodelling activity measured by undecalcified iliac crest biopsy, there is a significant correlation with the histological parameters reflecting bone formation but not with those reflecting resorption, both in the trabecular bone and the cortico-endosteal envelope (Brown et al, 1984, 1987; Podenphant et al, 1987). In most studies, serum TRAP, urinary hydroxyproline and crosslink excretion tend to be higher and more scattered than in age-matched controls. Recognizing this variable level of bone turnover might be important for choosing the optimal therapy. Indeed, a recent study has shown that the subgroup of osteoporotic patients with high bone turnover—characterized by increased whole body retention of labelled bisphosphonates, osteocalcin and hydroxyproline—showed a significant increase in spinal bone mineral density after 1 year of calcitonin therapy. In contrast, those with a low turnover had no increase in bone mass despite the same therapy (Civitelli et al, 1988). In women with vertebral osteoporosis treated with transdermal oestradiol, estimation of bone resorption with D-Pyr has been found to be useful in identifying women who are responding to the therapy (Eastell et al, 1990).

Finally, biochemical markers should be useful to monitor patients on chronic corticosteroid therapy, which inhibits osteoblastic activity, as reflected by a subnormal serum osteocalcin level (Reid et al, 1986; Garrel et al, 1988).

BONE TURNOVER IN ELDERLY WOMEN WITH HIP FRACTURE

Despite the importance of hip fracture as a major health problem, few studies have been devoted to potential bone turnover abnormalities in these patients. Histological studies suggest increased bone resorption as a consequence of secondary hyperparathyroidism. Increased serum alkaline phosphatase activity is thought to reflect the occurrence of osteomalacia, which is not uncommon in Europe in the elderly. Serum osteocalcin and urinary hydroxyproline have been reported to be either low or normal (Thompson et al, 1989; Delmi et al, 1990), but the acute changes in body fluids—and perhaps in bone turnover—related to the trauma might obscure the subtle changes due to bone remodelling. In a large group of patients studied immediately after hip fractures we have found increased urinary crosslinks excretion and decreased serum osteocalcin levels compared with age-matched healthy elderly (Akesson et al, 1990). Increased bone resorption and decreased bone formation might be an important determinant of the low bone mass which characterizes patients with hip fracture (Akesson et al, 1990) and should be further evaluated by prospective studies.

CONCLUSION

There is not as yet an ideal marker of bone formation, but circulating osteocalcin is the most satisfactory at the present time. New developments include the use of sheep and human osteocalcin as immunogens, and various monoclonal antibodies for measuring specifically the intact molecule (sandwich assay) but also for identifying fragments of osteocalcin released during resorption, if any. Unresolved questions include the volume of distribution of osteocalcin, its concentration in various compartments of bone (cortical versus trabecular), its metabolic clearance in humans, and the relative fractions of newly synthesized osteocalcin incorporated into the matrix or released into the circulation, which may vary in some diseases. The specific measurement of bone alkaline phosphatase and the assay of procollagen fragments and other non-collagenous bone-related proteins will in the future allow a more precise assessment of the complex osteoblastic dysfunction which occurs in osteoporosis. Finding a sensitive and specific marker of resorption is a challenge because all constituents of bone matrix are likely to be degraded into minute peptides during osteoclastic bone resorption. The measurement of pyridinium crosslinks, and to a lesser extent of TRAP by a bone-specific monoclonal antibody, are the most tangible improvements in this area, but these markers still need to be further validated. It should be remembered, however, that circulating markers reflect the activity of the whole skeleton, including cortical and trabecular bone, and depend both on the number and the activity of bone cells. Conversely, bone histomorphometry is limited to a small area of the trabecular envelope but allows the detection of a specific defect at the cellular level. These differences should be kept in mind, as there is growing evidence that bone mass and bone turnover of osteoporotic patients before and during treatment varies in different appendicular/axial and cortical/trabecular compartments. Therefore, biochemical markers, bone histomorphometry and bone densitometry should be seen as complementary techniques to investigate osteoporosis.

SUMMARY

The non-invasive assessment of bone turnover has received increasing attention over the past few years because of the need for sensitive markers in the clinical investigation of osteoporosis. Markers of bone formation include serum total and bone-specific alkaline phosphatase, serum osteocalcin, and measurement of serum type I collagen extension peptides. Assessment of bone resorption can be achieved with measurement of urinary hydroxyproline, urinary excretion of the pyridinium crosslinks (Pyr and D-Pyr), and by measurement of plasma TRAP activity. For the screening of bone turnover in women at the menopause, and for the assessment of the level of bone turnover in elderly women with vertebral osteoporosis, serum osteocalcin and urinary Pyr and D-Pyr appear to be the most sensitive markers so far. Programmes combining bone mass measurement and assessment of bone turnover in women at the time of the menopause have been developed in an attempt to improve the assessment of the risk for osteoporosis. Efforts are being made to develop more convenient assays and to identify other markers of bone turnover. In the future a battery of various specific markers is likely to improve the assessment of the complex aspects of bone metabolism, especially in osteoporosis.

Acknowledgements

I am grateful to Dr J. Brown, B. Demiaux, B. Fournier, L. Malaval and D. Uebelhart for their contributions, and to E. Gineyts and B. Merle for excellent technical assistance.

REFERENCES

Akesson K, Vergnaud P, Gineyts E et al (1990) Biochemical evidence for decreased bone formation and increased bone resorption in women with hip fracture. In Christiansen C & Overgaard K (eds) *Osteoporosis 1990*, vol. 1, pp 362–363. Copenhagen: Osteopress.

Bataille R, Delmas P & Sany J (1987) Serum bone gla-protein in multiple myeloma. *Cancer* 59: 329–334.

Black D, Duncan A & Robins SP (1988) Quantitative analysis of the pyridinium crosslinks of collagen in urine using ion-paired reversed-phase high-performance liquid chromatography. *Annals of Clinical Biochemistry* 169: 197–203.

Brown JP, Delmas PD, Malaval L et al (1984) Serum bone gla-protein: A specific marker for bone formation in postmenopausal osteoporosis. *Lancet* i: 1091–1093.

Brown JP, Delmas PD, Arlot M et al (1987) Active bone turnover of the cortico-endosteal envelope in postmenopausal osteoporosis. *Journal of Clinical Endocrinology and Metabolism* 64: 954–959.

Chenu C & Delmas PD (1990) Radioimmunoassay for bone sialoprotein: assessment of circulating levels. In Cohn DV et al (eds) *Calcium Regulation and Bone Metabolism*, International Congress Series 886, p 247. New York, Amsterdam: Elsevier.

Civitelli R, Gonnelli S, Zacchei F et al (1988) Bone turnover in postmenopausal osteoporosis. Effect of calcitonin treatment. *Journal of Clinical Investigation* 82: 1268–1274.

Colwell A, Eastell R, Assiri AMA & Russell RGG (1990) Effect of diet on deoxypyrinoline excretion. In Christiansen C & Overgaard K (eds) *Osteoporosis 1990*, vol. 2, pp 520–591. Copenhagen: Osteopress.

Delmas PD (1988) Biochemical markers of bone turnover in osteoporosis. In Riggs BL & Melton LJ (eds) *Osteoporosis: Etiology, Diagnosis and Management*, p 297. New York: Raven Press.

Delmas PD (1990) Biochemical markers of bone turnover for the clinical assessment of metabolic disease. *Endocrinology and Metabolism Clinics of North America* 19: 1–18.

Delmas PD, Stenner D, Wahner HW et al (1983) Serum bone gla-protein increases with aging in normal women: implications for the mechanism of age-related bone loss. *Journal of Clinical Investigation* 71: 1316–1321.

Delmas PD, Malaval L, Arlot MD & Meunier PJ (1985) Serum bone gla-protein compared to bone histomorphometry in endocrine diseases. *Bone* 6: 329–341.

Delmas PD, Demiaux B, Malaval L et al (1986) Serum bone gla-protein (osteocalcin) in primary hyperparathyroidism and in malignant hypercalcemia. Comparison with bone histomorphometry. *Journal of Clinical Investigation* 77: 985–991.

Delmas PD, Lacroze S, Chapuy MC & Malaval L (1987) Circadian rhythm in serum bone gla-protein (sBGP) concentration in the human: correlation with serum 1,25 dihydroxy-vitamin D (1,25(OH)$_2$D). In Cohn DV, Martin TJ & Meunier PJ (eds) *Calcium Regulation and Bone Metabolism*, International Congress Series 735, p 593. New York, Amsterdam: Elsevier.

Delmi M, Rapin CH, Bengoa JM et al (1990) Dietary supplementation in elderly patients with fractured neck of femur. *Lancet* 335: 1013–1016.

Duda RJ, O'Brien JF, Katzmann JA et al (1988) Concurrent assays of circulating bone gla-protein and bone alkaline phosphatase: effects of sex, age, and metabolic bone disease. *Journal of Clinical Endocrinology and Metabolism* 66: 951–957.

Eastell R, Delmas PD, Hodgson SF et al (1988) Bone formation rate in older normal women: concurrent assessment with bone histomorphometry, calcium kinetics and biochemical markers. *Journal of Clinical Endocrinology and Metabolism* 67: 741–748.

Eastell R, Colwell A, Assiri AMA et al (1990) Prediction of response to estrogen therapy using urine deoxypyridinoline. *Journal of Bone and Mineral Research* 5: S275.

Eyre DR (1987) Collagen crosslinking amino-acids. *Methods in Enzymology* 144: 115–139.

Eyre DR, Koob TJ & Van Ness KP (1984) Quantitation of hydroxypyridinium crosslinks in collagen by high-performance liquid chromatography. *Annals of Clinical Biochemistry* **137**: 380–388.

Eyre DR, Dickson IR & Van Ness KP (1988) Collagen cross-linking in human bone and articular cartilage. Age-related changes in the content of mature hydroxypyridinium residues. *Biochemical Journal* **252**: 495–500.

Farley JR, Chesnut CJ & Baylink DJ (1981) Improved method for quantitative determination in serum alkaline phosphatase of skeletal origin. *Clinical Chemistry* **27**: 2002–2007.

Fournier B, Gineyts E & Delmas PD (1989) Evidence that free gamma-carboxyglutamic acid circulates in serum. *Clinica Chimica Acta* **182**: 173–182.

Garrel DR, Delmas PD, Welsh C et al (1988) Effect of moderate physical training on prednisone-induced protein wasting: a study of whole bone and bone protein metabolism. *Metabolism: Clinical and Experimental* **37**: 257–262.

Gundberg C & Weinstein RS (1986) Multiple immunoreactive forms in uremic serum. *Journal of Clinical Investigation* **77**: 1762–1767.

Gundberg CM, Lian JM, Gallop PM et al (1983) Urinary gamma-carboxyglutamic acid and serum osteocalcin as bone markers: studies in osteoporosis and Paget's disease. *Journal of Clinical Endocrinology and Metabolism* **57**: 1221–1225.

Hill CS & Wolfert RL (1989) The preparation of monoclonal antibodies which react preferentially with human bone alkaline phosphatase and not liver alkaline phosphatase. *Clinica Chimica Acta* **186**: 315–320.

Johansen JS, Riss BJ, Delmas PD et al (1988) Plasma BGP: an indicator of spontaneous bone loss and effect of estrogen treatment in postmenopausal women. *European Journal of Clinical Investigation* **18**: 191–195.

Kivirikko KI (1983) Excretion of urinary hydroxyproline peptide in the assessment of bone collagen deposition and resorption. In Frame B & Potts JT Jr (eds) *Clinical Disorders of Bone and Mineral Metabolism*, pp 105–107. Amsterdam: Excerpta Medica.

Kraenzlin ME, Mohan S & Baylink DJ (1989) Development of a radioimmunoassay for the N-terminal type I procollagen: potential use to assess bone formation. *European Journal of Clinical Investigation* **19**: A86.

Kraenzlin M, Lau KHW, Liang et al (1990) Development of an immunoassay for human serum osteoclastic tartrate-resistant acid phosphatase. *Journal of Clinical Endocrinology and Metabolism* **71**: 442–451.

Li CY, Chuda RA, Lam WKW et al (1973) Acid phosphatase in human plasma. *Journal of Laboratory and Clinical Medicine* **82**: 446–460.

Lian JB & Gundberg CM (1988) Osteocalcin. Biochemical considerations and clinical applications. *Clinical Orthopaedics and Related Research* **226**: 267–291.

Lowry M, Hall DE & Brosnan JJ (1985) Hydroxyproline metabolism by the rat kidney: distribution of renal enzymes of hydroxyproline catabolism and renal conversion of hydroxyproline to glycine-and serine. *Metabolism* **39**: 955.

Malaval L, Fournier B & Delmas PD (1987) Radioimmunoassay for osteonectin. Concentrations in bone, nonmineralized tissues and blood. *Journal of Bone and Mineral Research* **2**: 457–465.

Malaval L, Darbouret B, Preaudat C et al (1988) Monoclonal antibody recognizing osteonectin from bone but not from platelet. *Journal of Bone and Mineral Research* **3**: S208.

Minkin C (1982) Bone acid phosphatase: Tartrate-resistant acid phosphatase as a marker of osteoclast function. *Calcified Tissue International* **34**: 285–290.

Moro L, Mucelli RSP, Gazzarrini C et al (1988a) Urinary β-1-galactosyl-O-hydroxylysine (GH) as a marker of collagen turnover of bone. *Calcified Tissue International* **42**: 87–90.

Moro L, Modricky C, Rovis L et al (1988b) Determination of galactosyl hydroxylysine in urine as a mean for the identification of osteoporotic women. *Bone and Mineral* **3**: 271–276.

Moss DW (1982) Alkaline phosphatase isoenzymes. *Clinical Chemistry* **28**: 2007–2016.

Nielsen HK, Brixen K, Bouillon R & Mosekilde L (1990) Changes in biochemical markers of osteoblastic activity during the menstrual cycle. *Journal of Clinical Endocrinology and Metabolism* **70**: 1431.

Parfitt AM, Simon LS, Villanueva AR et al (1987) Procollagen type I Carboxyterminal extension peptide in serum as a marker of collagen biosynthesis in bone. Correlation with iliac bone formation rates and comparison with total alkaline phosphatase. *Journal of Bone and Mineral Research* **2**: 427–436.

Piedra C, Torres R, Rapado A et al (1989) Serum tartrate resistant acid phosphatase and bone mineral content in postmenopausal osteoporosis. *Calcified Tissue International* **45**: 58–60.

Podenphant J, Johansen JS, Thomsen K et al (1987) Bone turnover in spinal osteoporosis. *Journal of Bone and Mineral Research* **2**: 497–503.

Price PA (1987) Vitamin K-dependent bone proteins. In Cohn DV, Martin TJ & Meunier PJ (eds) *Calcium Regulation and Bone Metabolism. Basic and Clinical Aspects*, vol. 9, pp 419–426. New York, Amsterdam: Elsevier.

Price PA, Parthemore JG & Deftos LJ (1980) New biochemical marker for bone metabolism. *Journal of Clinical Investigation* **66**: 878–883.

Price PA, Williamson MK & Lothringer JW (1981) Origin of vitamin K-dependent bone protein found in plasma and its clearance by kidney and bone. *Journal of Biological Chemistry* **256**: 12760–12766.

Prockop OJ & Kivirikko KI (1968) Hydroxyproline and the metabolism of collagen. In Gould BS (ed.) *Treatise on Collagen*, vol. 2, pp 215–246. New York: Academic Press.

Prockop DJ, Kivirikko KI, Tuderman K et al (1979) The biosynthesis of collagen and its disorders. *New England Journal of Medicine* **301**: 13–23.

Reid IR, Chapman GE, Fraser TRC et al (1986) Low serum osteocalcin levels in glucocorticoid-treated asthmatics. *Journal of Clinical Endocrinology and Metabolism* **62**: 379–383.

Simon LS & Krane SM (1983) Procollagen extension peptides as markers of collagen synthesis. In Frame B & Potts JJ Jr (eds) *Clinical Disorders of Bone and Mineral Metabolism*, pp 108–111. Amsterdam: Excerpta Medica.

Slemenda C, Hui SL, Longcope C et al (1987) Sex steroids and bone mass. A study of changes about the time of menopause. *Journal of Clinical Investigation* **80**: 1261–1269.

Stenner DD, Tracy RP, Riggs BL et al (1986) Human platelets contain and secrete osteonectin, a major protein of mineralized bone. *Proceedings of the National Academy of Sciences of the USA* **83**: 6892–6896.

Stepan JJ, Silinkova-Malkova E, Havrenek T et al (1983) Relationship of plasma tartrate-resistant acid phosphatase to the bone isoenzyme of serum alkaline phosphatase in hyperparathyroidism. *Clinica Chimica Acta* **133**: 189–200.

Stepan JJ, Pospichal J, Presl J et al (1987) Bone loss and biochemical indices of bone remodeling in surgically induced postmenopausal women. *Bone* **8**: 279–284.

Taylor et al (1990) Partial characterization of a novel growth factor from the blood of women with preeclampsia. *Journal of Clinical Endocrinology and Metabolism* **70**: 1285–1291.

Thompson SP, White DA, Hosking DJ, Wilton TJ & Pawley E (1989) Changes in osteocalcin after femoral neck fracture. *Annals of Clinical Biochemistry* **26**: 487–491.

Thomsen K, Rodbro P & Christiansen C (1987) Bone turnover determined by urinary excretion of [^{99m}Tc]-disphosphonate in the prediction of postmenopausal bone loss. *Bone and Mineral* **2**: 125–131.

Tracy RP, Andrianorivo A, Riggs BL & Mann KG (1990) Comparison of monoclonal and polyclonal antibody-based immunoassays for osteocalcin. A study of sources of variation in assay results. *Journal of Bone and Mineral Research* **5**: 451–461.

Uebelhart D, Gineyts E, Chapuy MC & Delmas PD (1990) Urinary excretion of pyridinium crosslinks: a new marker of bone resorption in metabolic bone disease. *Bone and Mineral* **8**: 87–96.

Uebelhart D, Schlemmer A, Johansen J, Gineyts E, Christiansen C & Delmas PD (1991) Effect of menopause and hormone replacement therapy on the urinary excretion of pyridinium crosslinks. *Journal of Clinical Endocrinology and Metabolism* **72**: 367–373.

4

Biochemical markers—a new approach for identifying those at risk of osteoporosis

BENTE JUEL RIIS

CALCIUM METABOLISM AND BIOCHEMICAL MARKERS

In the perimenopausal years, calcium metabolism changes considerably (Nilas and Christiansen, 1987). Primarily, bone resorption increases from 280 to 470 mg/day (Heaney et al, 1987) and, secondarily, bone formation (expressed as the accretion rate) increases from 230 to 380 mg/day. This increased bone turnover results in a negative calcium balance of approximately 50 mg/day, which is reflected in an increased urinary calcium output. However, the 50 mg daily negative calcium balance cannot be detected within a reasonable period of time by the methods currently available for measuring bone mass.

Bone metabolism may be studied directly using bone biopsies, but this method is invasive and determines qualitative rather than quantitative parameters. The small biopsy sample may, furthermore, not be representative of the entire skeleton. Study of calcium kinetics is expensive and time consuming, and requires administration of radioactive isotopes. For quantitative determinations the biochemical indices of bone turnover have therefore proved to be of value.

The concentration of serum alkaline phosphatase has been used as a marker of bone formation and the urinary excretion of calcium and hydroxyproline as markers of bone resorption (Lauffenburger et al, 1977). Although not specific for bone metabolism, these parameters have been of appreciable value in both calcium metabolism research and in the clinical situation.

Recently, bone gla-protein (BGP), also known as osteocalcin, has been identified and purified. BGP is a small non-collagenous protein synthesized predominantly by osteoblasts. It is incorporated into the organic matrix of bone; however, a fraction of neosynthesized BGP is released into the circulation where it can be measured by radioimmunoassay (Price and Nishimoto, 1980). Numerous studies have demonstrated that BGP is specific for bone, and that serum concentrations provide a measure of bone formation (Brown et al, 1987; Johansen et al, 1988).

New markers are currently being developed. Type I collagen accounts for more than 90% of the organic substance of bone (Burgeson, 1988). It is synthesized by osteoblasts as type I procollagen, which at both ends has two

---

Baillière's Clinical Obstetrics and Gynaecology—
Vol. 5, No. 4, December 1991
ISBN 0–7020–1548–2

relatively long sequences known as the amino acid carboxyterminal pro-peptides of type I procollagen (Prockop et al, 1979). The carboxyterminal propeptide (PICP) is removed in the extracellular space before the collagen molecule is incorporated into the bone matrix. PICP has thus been proposed as a potential marker of bone formation (Parfitt et al, 1987; Hassager et al, 1990).

Pyridinoline (Pyr) and deoxypyridinoline (D-Pyr) are crosslinks of the mature form of the collagen. Pyr is present in type I collagen of bone and in type II collagen of cartilage, but it is absent in skin collagen. D-Pyr has, on the other hand, only been found in type I collagen of bone, and has not been observed in cartilage, tendon, skin or cornea (Eyre, 1987). The crosslinks are released during collagen breakdown and are excreted unmetabolized in the urine. Pyr and especially D-Pyr are thus potential markers of bone resorption (Uebelhart et al, 1990).

γ-Carboxyglutamic acid (gla) is an amino acid formed by post-translational modification of glutamic acid. It primarily originates from the vitamin K-dependent clotting factors and from non-collageneous proteins of bone. Free gla circulates in serum, and it has been suggested that it may reflect the degradation of gla-containing bone proteins (Parfitt et al, 1987; Fournier et al, 1988, 1989).

Osteoporosis is one of the most significant metabolic bone diseases. It affects millions of people, especially women, throughout the world (Table 1). Fortunately, osteoporosis is preventable, but to take efficient preventive measures it is necessary that the women at risk of osteoporosis are identified. The biochemical markers of bone turnover may be important tools in this diagnostic procedure.

Table 1. Expected number of cases of hip fractures in England and Wales in 1996, 2006 and 2016 (a) assuming current age- and sex-specific incidence rates continue unchanged and (b) assuming the present increasing trend continues.

(a) Assuming 1985 age- and sex-specific rates continue unchanged:

	1985	1996	2006	2016
No. of cases	46 000	54 000	58 000	60 000

(b) Assuming 1985 age- and sex-specific rates double between 1985 and 2016 (i.e. the present trend continues):

	1985	1996	2006	2016
No. of cases	46 000	71 000	94 000	117 000

BONE MASS AND BONE LOSS

The bone mass at, for example, the age of 70 years is theoretically determined by the peak bone mass and the loss of bone after the peak bone mass has been attained. Both men and women experience bone loss after skeletal maturity (Geusens et al, 1986; Thomsen et al, 1986). This bone loss may be aggravated by several factors (Table 2), including certain drugs

Table 2. Risk factors for osteoporosis.

Genetic factors:
White and Asian women
Thin or petite women
Familial history of osteoporosis
Early menopause, premenopausal states of oestrogen deficiency
Lifestyle factors:
Prolonged periods of inadequate calcium nutrition
Cigarette smoking
Alcohol abuse
Sedentary lifestyle
Endocrine factors:
Oestrogen deficiency
Glucocorticoid excess
Primary hyperparathyroidism
Hyperthyroidism
Multiple myeloma

(steroids), certain diseases (thyrotoxicosis), heredity, cigarettes, alcohol, coffee, sedentary lifestyle and low calcium intake. By far the most important factor is, however, oestrogen deficiency. The fact that men and women at maturity seem to be provided equally with bone mass in terms of mechanical resistance, and that osteoporosis is so much more common in women, indicates that postmenopausal bone loss plays an important role in the pathogenesis of symptomatic osteoporosis. The woman who passes through the menopause with a 'low' bone mass will eventually develop symptomatic osteoporosis irrespective of whether her postmenopausal bone loss is 'slow' or 'fast'. As a result, this woman is a candidate to receive preventive therapy.

A woman passing through the menopause with a 'normal' or 'high' bone mass and who experiences an accelerated postmenopausal bone loss may eventually have a bone mass that predisposes to fractures. Furthermore, an unphysiologically fast bone loss may predispose to fracture, even without reaching a 'low' bone mass. This is supported by the finding of a group of postmenopausal women with spinal crush fractures and a relatively normal spinal bone mass (Lyritis, 1986). This type of osteoporosis, which may correspond to type I osteoporosis as defined by Riggs and Melton (1983), may be the result of quick bone loss and a lack of adjustment of the skeleton to tolerating the usual mechanical loads. This may include impairment of bone quality (Heaney, 1987). The importance of such a 'relative' low bone mass (i.e. relative to peak bone mass) remains to be settled.

THE BIOCHEMICAL APPROACH

In 1984 we proposed the biochemical approach for identifying the fast bone losers, and the data were later published (Christiansen et al, 1987). The idea was generated by the observation that, in a large group of early post-menopausal women who were followed up with bone mass measurements

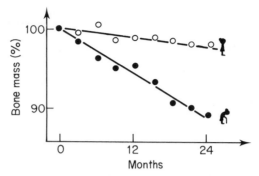

Figure 1. Bone mass as a function of time in two age-matched early postmenopausal women. One woman was losing bone at a rate of 1% per year and the other at 5% per year. It would be expected that fractures would occur more frequently with the more rapid rate of loss. From C. Christiansen, with permission.

for 2 years, some lost considerably more bone mass than others (Figure 1). The two groups were similar in almost all aspects (such as initial bone mineral content, smoking habits, parity, etc.), but differed significantly in mass of fat, serum oestrogen concentrations and in biochemical estimates of bone turnover. The application of these parameters in a cut-off technique or a multiple regression analysis yielded the same type of information (Christiansen et al, 1987): 20% of the women could be characterized correctly as fast or slow bone losers, whereas 20% were false negative or false positive.

We also substituted body weight (fat mass (FM)/cm = body weight/ height) with plasma BGP (pBGP) in order to see whether the model could be improved. Table 3 gives the diagnostic validity of the two studies using either FM/cm or pBGP. It appears that pBGP improved the diagnostic validity (Christiansen et al, 1990).

Table 3. Diagnostic validity including fat mass (FM) or BGP with the individual parameters either as absolute values or as a percentage of premenopausal values.

	Absolute values		% of premenopausal values	
	FM*	BGP†	FM*	BGP†
PV positive	0.67	0.70	0.68	0.75
PV negative	0.84	0.87	0.82	0.81
Sensitivity	0.64	0.73	0.59	0.59
Specificity	0.85	0.85	0.88	0.91
Slope	1.00	1.00	1.00	1.00
Intercept	0.00	0.00	0.00	0.00
r values	0.72	0.76	0.72	0.76
SEE values	1.01	0.94	1.01	0.94

PV, predictive value.
* FM/cm, alkaline phosphatase, urinary calcium and urinary hydroxy-proline.
† BGP, alkaline phosphatase, urinary calcium and urinary hydroxy-proline.

DISCUSSION

The present data demonstrate that it is possible to select just around the menopause women who are 'fast bone losers' and who therefore probably will be particularly at risk for developing fractures in the future. Although the rate of bone loss changes during life, i.e. it accelerates around the menopause and levels off 8–10 years later, we believe that a 'fast bone loser' will always continue losing bone faster than her 'normal bone loser' counterpart. This is supported by the very small variation around the individual woman's regression line (SEE% = 0.37–3.03; mean ± 1sp = 42 ± 0.51). Although the bone mass was measured locally in the forearm, we have previously demonstrated that this area correlates well with total body calcium, which support the diagnostic validity of the model. It has been suggested that trabecular bone (e.g. in the spine) is decalcified more rapidly than cortical bone (e.g. in the forearm). A 'fast loser' in the forearm would thus be even more a 'fast loser' in the spine. It is unlikely that a woman could be a 'fast loser' in the forearm but not in the spine.

The present studies provide a simple and valid model for the identification of women at risk for developing osteoporosis. The ideal screening procedure would be one bone mass measurement and one estimation of future bone loss at the time of the menopause.

REFERENCES

Brown JP, Delmas PD, Arlot M et al (1987) Active bone turnover of the cortico-endosteal envelope in postmenopausal osteoporosis. *Journal of Clinical Endocrinology and Metabolism* **64:** 954–959.

Burgeson RE (1988) New collagens, new concepts. *Annual Review of Cell Biology* **4:** 551–577.

Christiansen C, Riis BJ & Rødbro P (1987) Prediction of rapid bone loss in postmenopausal women. *Lancet* **i:** 1105–1107.

Christiansen C, Riis BJ & Rødbro P (1990) Screening procedure for women at risk of developing postmenopausal osteoporosis. *Osteoporosis International* **1:** 35–40.

Eyre D (1987) Collagen crosslinking amino-acids. *Methods in Enzymology* **144:** 115–139.

Fournier B, Gineyts E & Delmas PD (1988) Measurement of free gamma-carboxyglutamic acid in serum: A new marker of bone turnover. *Journal of Bone and Mineral Research* **3:** 402 (abstract).

Fournier B, Gineyts E & Delmas PD (1989) Evidence that free gamma carboxyglutamic acid circulates in serum. *Clinica Chimica Acta* **182:** 173–183.

Geusens P, Dequeker J, Verstraeten A & Nijs J (1986) Age-, sex- and menopause related changes of vertebral and peripheral bone: population study using dual and single photon absorptiometry and radiogrammetry. *Journal of Nuclear Medicine* **27:** 1540–1549.

Hassager C, Jensen LT, Johansen JS et al (1990) The carboxy-terminal propeptide of type I procollagen in serum as a marker of bone formation: The effect of anabolic steroids and female sex hormones. *Metabolism: Clinical and Experimental* **39:** 1167–1169.

Heaney RP (1987) Qualitative factors in osteoporosis fracture: the state of the question. In Christiansen C, Johansen JS & Riis BJ (eds) *Osteoporosis 1987.* Proceedings of the International Symposium on Osteoporosis, Aalborg, Denmark, vol. 1, pp 281–287. Copenhagen: Osteopress.

Heaney RP, Recker RR & Saville PD (1987) Menopausal changes in calcium balance performance. *Journal of Laboratory and Clinical Medicine* **92:** 953–963.

Johansen JS, Riis BJ, Delmas PD et al (1988) Plasma BGP: An indicator of spontaneous bone loss and effect of estrogen treatment in postmenopausal women. *European Journal of Clinical Investigation* **18**: 191–195.

Lauffenburger T, Olah AJ, Dambacher MA, Guncaga J, Lentner C & Haas HG (1977) Bone remodeling and calcium metabolism: A correlated histomorphometric, calcium kinetic, and biochemical study in patients with osteoporosis and Paget's disease. *Metabolism: Clinical and Experimental* **26**: 589–606.

Lyritis GP (1986) Classification of the osteoporotic vertebral fractures. *European Journal of Clinical Investigation* **19**: A85.

Nilas L & Christiansen C (1987) Bone mass and its relationship to age and the menopause. *Journal of Clinical Endocrinology and Metabolism* **65**: 697–702.

Parfitt AM, Simon LS, Villanueva AR & Krane SM (1987) Procollagen type I carboxy-terminal extension peptide in serum as a marker of collagen biosynthesis in bone. Correlation with iliac bone formation rates a comparison with total alkaline phosphatase. *Journal of Bone and Mineral Research* **2**: 427–436.

Price PA & Nishimoto SK (1980) Radioimmunoassay for the vitamin K-dependent protein of bone and its discovery in plasma. *Proceedings of the National Academy of Sciences of the USA* **77**: 2234–2238.

Prockop DJ, Kivirikko KI, Tuderman L & Guzman AN (1979) The biosynthesis of collagen and its disorders. *New England Journal of Medicine* **309**: 13–23.

Riggs BL & Melton LJ (1983) Evidence for two distinct syndromes of involutional osteoporosis. *American Journal of Medicine* **75**: 899–901.

Thomsen K, Gotfredsen A & Christiansen C (1986) Is postmenopausal bone loss an age-related phenomenon? *Calcified Tissue International* **39**: 123–127.

Uebelhart D, Gineyts E, Chapyu M-C & Delmas PD (1990) Urinary excretion of pyridinium crosslinks: A new marker of bone resorption in metabolic bone disease. *Bone and Mineral* **8**: 87–96.

5

Why do oestrogens prevent bone loss?

ROBERT LINDSAY

As is reviewed elsewhere in this issue, in addition to the loss of mass that occurs in the skeleton as osteoporosis develops, significant architectural alterations also occur. The most serious of these, for cancellous bone at least, is the complete loss of trabecular elements. As far as is known it is not possible for any pharmacological agent to stimulate the synthesis of new bone without an existing template. Even if agents that will reconstitute trabeculae can be developed, there is no guarantee that the architecture necessary to maintain skeletal status in the presence of normal stresses will be reconstituted. The likelihood is, therefore, that osteoporosis will be more effectively prevented than treated. Additionally, there is at present no therapeutic intervention that adequately deals with the changes in body configuration that occur after vertebral fracture. Although experimental surgical approaches are being investigated, there are no practical approaches to correcting the kyphosis and height loss that follows multiple vertebral crush fractures. In this chapter the effects of loss of ovarian function on the skeleton are reviewed, and the use of sex steroids in prevention and treatment are discussed. Because postmenopausal osteoporosis does not occur in a vacuum, of necessity other issues must be discussed, including, for example, calcium and exercise, but the discussion of such issues will be oriented around the primary problem of ovarian failure and its correction.

THE ROLE OF THE MENOPAUSE

Albright originally drew attention to the relationship between oestrogen lack, due either to early menopause or oophorectomy, and osteoporosis, and also suggested that oestrogen therapy could be used in the treatment of this condition (Albright et al, 1941; Albright, 1947). Albright hypothesized that oestrogens were anabolic agents and acted on osteoblasts (Albright, 1947), a feature which did not seem to be correct in subsequent studies. In a publication following some of Albright's original patients, Henneman and Wallach (1957) demonstrated that oestrogen-treated osteoporotic patients ceased to lose height. During the ensuing 20 years there were several

Baillière's Clinical Obstetrics and Gynaecology—
Vol. 5, No. 4, December 1991
ISBN 0–7020–1548–2

uncontrolled studies of the effects of oestrogen, and the relationship between the sex hormones and the skeleton continued to be debated (Lindsay, 1984; Draper, 1985; Murrills et al, 1990). The development of techniques that enabled easy reliable measurement of skeletal mass has now for the first time allowed controlled evaluation of the effects of oestrogen on bone loss after failure of the ovaries.

The gradual decline of ovarian function is a ubiquitous occurrence among women. The human species is, for all practical purposes, the only animal species to live sufficiently long to undergo a natural menopause. In particular, the female of the human species can expect to live almost one-third of her life after the complete cessation of ovarian function (almost 30 years). Thus, if loss of the endocrine secretion of the ovary has an adverse impact on health, it would only be likely to be manifest in the human.

Cross-sectional studies of bone mass tend to show an inflection downward coincident with the decline in ovarian function (Meema, 1966; Mazess and Mather, 1974; Aloia et al, 1978; Heaney et al, 1978a, b; Riggs et al, 1981; Firooznia et al, 1986; Riis et al, 1987; Genant et al, 1988, 1989; Mazess and Wahner, 1988; Stevenson et al, 1989; Lindsay et al, 1991). Studies on calcium balance have indicated that this is a real loss of bone tissue that results from a variety of factors that change across the menopause (Heaney et al, 1978a, b). There is an increase in the movement of calcium into and out of bone, thought to represent an increase in the activation of new remodelling sites. At each remodelling site bone is first resorbed and later replaced with new bone tissue. Within each unit there needs to be balance. Among premenopausal women this balance is nearly achieved, but in the postmenopausal state there is excess bone resorption, and thus a negative balance at each remodelling unit (Albright, 1947). The currently available data suggest that the osteoclast population resorb more bone and, although osteoblasts also synthesize more new bone at each remodelling site, the teams of osteoblasts fail to make sufficient new tissue to competely repair the cavity created by the osteoclasts (Albright et al, 1940). Thus there is a negative balance at each site, with consequent irreversible loss of tissue, since once the remodelling process is completed at that site there is no mechanism for increasing the amount of bone until remodelling begins again. The increased avidity of the osteoclasts results in penetration of trabecular units in cancellous bone, and their eventual removal (Dempster et al, 1986). The loss of a template upon which to lay down new bone tissue is a major factor in the irreversibility of osteoporosis (Figure 1).

The consequence of these alterations is a reduction in skeletal mass that leads to increased risk of fracture (Johnston et al, 1989). The data suggest that those at greatest risk are those with the lowest bone mass when entering the point of increased loss, that is menopause. Consequently bone mass measurement can be used as an indicator of fracture risk (Slemenda et al, 1987b; Ross et al, 1988; Gardsell et al, 1989; Johnston et al, 1989). Measurement of the skeleton thus estimates one of the risk factors for fracture (i.e. low bone mass). This is analogous to the use of cholesterol or any composite of the circulating lipids in serum to estimate the risk of coronary heart disease or blood pressure for the risk of cerebrovascular accident. In fact if

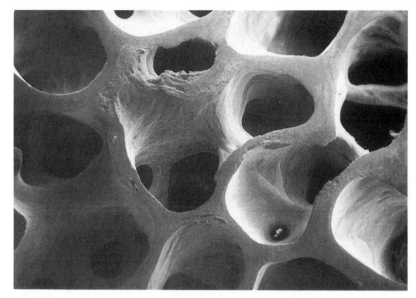

(a)

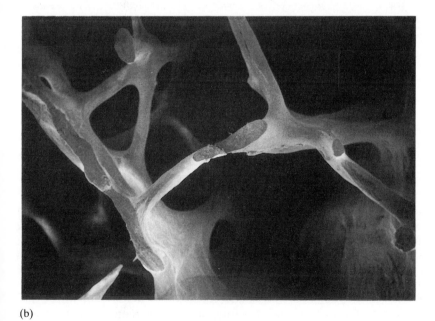

(b)

Figure 1.

one examines blood pressure or cholesterol in patients with cerebrovascular accident or myocardial infarction, overlaps are found with the 'normal' population (Hui et al, 1990). The relationship between fracture risk and bone mass is as strong or even stronger than the relationship between cholesterol and coronary heart disease. Several studies, perhaps not surprisingly, have demonstrated that baseline measurements of bone mass are predictive of the risk for future fracture (Slemenda et al, 1987b; Hui et al, 1988; Ross et al, 1988; Gardsell et al, 1989; Johnston et al, 1989) (Figure 2). Measurements of the skeleton should also be obtained when there is radiological evidence to support the diagnosis of osteoporosis, and thus to eliminate the possibility that trauma caused the abnormality. In this circumstance bone mass also allows evaluation of the severity of the problem.

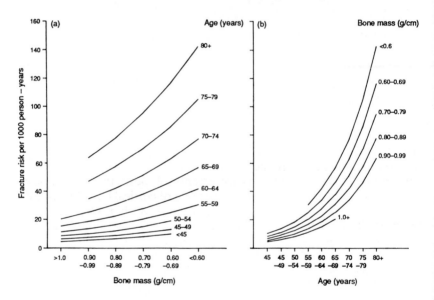

Figure 2. Estimated incidence of fracture as a function of age (a) and bone mass (b).

For the average 50-year-old woman the lifetime risk of fracture is about 15% (Cummings et al, 1989). For a woman with a bone mass at the upper end of the normal range the risk of a similar fracture is less than 2%, rising to 40% for those at the 5th percentile (Johnston et al, 1989). The data available thus far indicate that measurement can be made at any site and still be predictive of fractures of the appendicular skeleton. What is not clear is whether measurement of mass made, for example, in the spine will be more predictive of vertebral crush fractures than measurements made at other sites. Similar questions can be asked about measurements made at the femoral neck, which logically one might think would be more predictive for hip fractures.

A common misconception is that those at particular risk of osteoporosis can be identified by clinical observation (Johnston et al, 1989; Van Hemert et al, 1990). This has never been demonstrated in a prospective study. There is evidence that broad classifications can be used for population studies. However, the extraction of those so-called risk factors into the clinic for use with individual patients is difficult, and may in fact prove impossible. In part this results from the low power that each factor contributes to the multiple regression when risk factors are examined as predictors of either fracture or bone mass. In addition, the wide variety of the proposed components to risk mean that studies have mostly evaluated only a selection of them at any one time. Some of these risk factors may not be independent, for example smoking and obesity. Others may be important, such as glucocorticoid use, malabsorption and thyrotoxicosis, but are sufficiently rare in the population that is being evaluated that their very presence alone can dictate further investigation of skeletal status.

These clinical risk factors are not only poor predictors of fracture risk, but are also poor predictors of bone mass. Most studies indicate that 40% or less of the variance in bone mass in a population can be accounted for by a variety of risk factors (Aloia et al, 1978). This would result in less than 50% of patients being correctly stratified using broad stratification restrictions, which is clearly inadequate for clinical use. One unpublished study had more success with an algorithm for bone mass based on height, weight and age (Arnett et al, 1986), but independent confirmation of this is required.

Other approaches to the determination of those most at risk of fracture have included the use of biochemical markers of bone remodelling or oestrogen status to determine bone loss. In our early studies of this we demonstrated that multiple measurements of oestradiol and oestrone (monthly for 2 years) correlated with the rate of cortical bone loss (Lindsay et al, 1984a). However, the power of the relationship was insufficiently useful to allow identification of those losing bone at the most rapid rate either from single or multiple determinations of sex steroids in the serum. Others have confirmed that there is indeed a relationship between endogenous oestrogen supply and rate of bone loss among perimenopausal women (Albright et al, 1940), but again the biochemical measurements are generally not valuable for individual patients.

Within the past few years there has been increasing interest in biochemical markers for bone remodelling, and assays for several have become more generally available. Osteocalcin (bone gla-protein), which has become the best known of these markers, has been recognized as a product of osteoblasts that circulates in serum (Price et al, 1980). Since there is an increase in both formation and resorption after the menopause, measurement of this compound has been investigated to determine if it would be capable of identifying individuals with increased skeletal metabolism and therefore likely to be losing bone most rapidly. It can, in fact, be demonstrated that in mixed populations there is a relationship between osteocalcin concentrations in serum and bone formation rate (Delmas, 1988; F. Cosman et al, unpublished data) and osteocalcin levels do rise after the menopause. However, again it has proven difficult to translate results obtained on group data to individuals. Similar problems are found in the use of any other single market, including alkaline or acid phosphatase, or urinary calcium or hydroxyproline. The more recent markers of bone remodelling, including the pyridinium cross-links and assays for the pro-collagen extension peptides, have as yet been insufficiently evaluated for us to know if they solve the inherent problems in relating biochemical indicators to rates of bone loss in individual patients (Lindsay et al, 1990).

The most sophisticated approach to this problem of easy identification of those most rapidly losing bone mass has been that of Christiansen et al (1987, 1990), who evaluated rate of loss by a single photon absorptiometry and predicted rate of loss from the results of several features estimated at a single visit. The addition of fat mass (from height and weight), serum alkaline phosphatase and oestradiol, and urinary calcium and hydroxyproline allowed determination of rate of bone loss. However, r^2 was 0.5, which is insufficient for routine clinical use. Additionally the cost of multiple biochemical investigations may be prohibitive unless specially provided.

The mechanism for the bone loss that occurs after the menopause is not entirely clear. Since for many years oestrogens were not thought to have specific receptors on cells derived from bone, it was assumed that the effects must be indirect, probably mediated by those endocrine factors normally responsible for both calcium and mineral homeostasis, namely the parathyroid hormone/vitamin D/calcitonin axes. The demonstration that cells of the osteoblast lineage had specific oestrogen receptors has revived interest in a direct effect of oestrogen upon the skeleton (Eriksen et al, 1988; Komm et al, 1988). A summary of some of the effects of oestrogen are listed in Table 1. Although the results are somewhat conflicting, it appears likely that oestrogen does have direct effects on the biological responses of these cells (Gray et al, 1987, 1989; Ernst et al, 1988, 1989; Bankson et al, 1989; Fukayama and Tashjian, 1989; Schmid et al, 1989). In vivo, however, the specific effects of oestrogen are a reduction in the frequency with which new remodelling cycles are activated, and perhaps also some inhibition of osteoclast-mediated resorption (Steiniche et al, 1989). Since osteoblasts (at least those inactive osteoblasts normally lining the surface of bone between times of active remodelling) may be responsible for activation (Parfitt, 1988), alterations of their biological function in response to oestrogen

Table 1. Oestrogen effects on osteoblasts and osteoblast cell lines.

Author	Year	Cell line	Response	
Gray	1987	UMR-106	↓ Cell division:	↑ Alk. phos.
Gray	1989	UMR-106	↑ IGF-1, IGF-2	
Bankson	1989	UMR-106	Variable response in unrelated enzymes	
Ernst	1988	Rat calvarial	↑ Proliferation	↑ Procoll mRNA
Schmid	1989	Rat calvarial	↑ IGF-1	
Ernst	1989	Rat calvarial	↑ Proliferation	↑ IGF-1 procoll mRNA
Keeting	1991	hOB	No effect	
Gray	1987	ROS17/2.8	No effect	
Komm	1988	ROS17/2.8	↑ Gene trans TGF-B, Type I procollagen	
Fukuyama	1989	SaOS-2	↓ PTH stimulated adenylyl cyclase	
Watts	1989	HTB-96	No response	
		HTB-96 transfected	↓ Cell proliferation	

clearly could be a mechanism of reducing the activation frequency. The precise biological alterations required to effect this are not known. Potential local mediators include TGF-β, IGFs, TNF and interferons (Komm et al, 1988; Ernst et al, 1989; Gray et al, 1989; Schmid et al, 1989). Another proposed mechanism for the effects of sex steroids on the skeleton is the release of other local factors from cells in the marrow from the haemopoietic system (Pacifici et al, 1987). One group has described increased secretion of interleukin 1 from monocytes after the menopause, the effect being reversed by oestrogen (Pacifici et al, 1987, 1989). Interleukin 1 has been proposed as a stimulator of bone resorption (Gowen et al, 1983), although this effect is not seen in in vitro systems (Murrills et al, 1990). Finally it has been suggested that oestoclasts may have functional oestrogen receptors (Oursler et al, 1990), although biological responses of these cells are not seen at physiological concentrations of oestrogen (Arnett et al, 1986).

OESTROGENS

Most, if not all studies of oestrogens have indicated that adequate oestrogen therapy retards the rate of bone loss at all skeletal sites, cementing the causal relationship between ovarian failure and bone loss (Riggs et al, 1969; Aitken et al, 1973; Burch et al, 1974; Meema et al, 1975; Lindsay et al, 1976, 1978b, 1980, 1984b; Horsman et al, 1977; Nachtigall et al, 1979; Cann et al, 1980; Christiansen et al, 1980; Christiansen and Rodbro, 1983, 1984; Al-Azzawi et al, 1987; Ettinger et al, 1987; Riis et al, 1987; Civitelli et al, 1988; Lindsay and Tohme, 1990; Stevenson et al, 1990). Measurement of peripheral cortical bone indicated that adequate oestrogen replacement was associated with complete conservation of bone mass for at least 10 years (Figure 3). The effects were evident in all women, even those in whom treatment had been delayed for 6 or more years after ovarian removal. However, because conservation of skeletal tissue was the outcome for all groups, those in whom treatment was delayed still had a lower bone mass than their peers who had been treated from the time of oophorectomy, even after 10 years of treatment.

Preservation of bone mass has been confirmed in women who have gone through a natural menopause and at all sites that have been measured, including the spine and hip, the major sites of importance for osteoporotic fracture. Consequently maintenance of total body calcium is also seen. The effects of oestrogen persist for as long as treatment is maintained, at least for 10 years and probably considerably longer, although most studies are only of 2 years' duration. When treatment is stopped bone loss begins again (Lindsay et al, 1978a; Christiansen et al, 1981). The rate at which this loss occurs appears to be parallel to the rate of bone loss immediately following ovarian removal in premenopausal women. Thus cessation of oestrogen therapy is a form of medical oophorectomy.

The skeleton does not appear to require any particular route of administration. Oestrogen given by mouth, by subcutaneous pellet (Garnett et al, 1990), percutaneously (Riis et al, 1987) and transdermally (Stevenson et al,

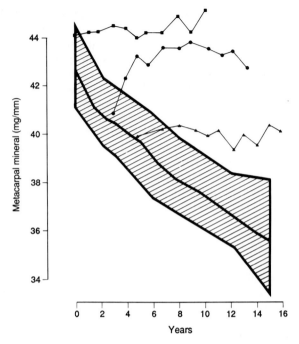

Figure 3. Long-term prevention of bone loss by oestrogen. The hatched area represents the placebo using (mean ±SD) a prospective controlled study in oophorectomized women. The three lines show the mean values only for three oestrogen-treated groups: treatment initiated at the time of oophorectomy (■), 3 years after (●) or 6 years after (▲) oophorectomy. Bone loss is prevented in all three situations. However, the earlier treatment is begun, the better the outcome, in terms of bone mass after 10 years of therapy.

1990) always reduces bone turnover and prevents bone loss in oestrogen-deprived women. The dose of oestrogen appears to be the factor that determines whether or not a skeletal effect will be seen. Circulating oestradiol levels of between 50 and 100 pg/ml appear to be sufficient to reduce bone turnover (Peacock and Selby, 1986). Such levels are seen after conjugated equine oestrogen (Premarin) 0.625 mg/day or transdermal oestrogen (Estraderm) 50 μg/day. Other available oestrogen preparations also provide sufficient oestrogen to reduce bone loss, and some, notably oestrogen pellets, provide higher concentrations in the circulation. These are currently not available in the USA but are used in Europe.

A considerable amount of epidemiological data has demonstrated that oestrogen intervention reduces the risk of fracture among older women (Hutchinson et al, 1979; Paganini-Hill et al, 1981; Kreiger et al, 1982; Kiel et al, 1987; Slemenda et al, 1987a). The reduction in the risk of hip fracture appears to be about 50%. The exact duration of therapy required to produce this effect is not clear. The only study which has attempted to evaluate this aspect suggested that a minimum of 5 years was required. In general the results seem better when oestrogen is introduced early in the postmenopausal period. A logical argument can be built on these results. It is clear from our scanning electon micrographs (Dempster et al, 1986) (Figure 1) that prevention of the alteration in trabecular architecture is likely to be important in fracture prevention. Since it appears that the major changes in architecture occur after menopausal loss of oestrogen, then early introduction of preventive therapy is likely to prove most successful. The argument about duration of therapy relies on the timing of the acceleration of bone loss and the age at which increased fractures begin to be a population problem. If we assume that the major acceleration of bone loss follows menopause, then it would start on average at age 50 years. If therapy were initiated at that point and continued for 5 years the acceleration of bone loss would be delayed for that period, i.e. until 55 years. The real increase in hip fracture begins at about 75 years, and the average life expectancy (for women in their 50s when the treatment being evaluated in these studies was begun) was about 80 years. If we assume that the delay in acceleration of bone loss by 5 years will result in an equal delay in hip fracture risk, then the main increase in hip fracture would be delayed until after 80 years and on a population basis would cease to be important.

Oestrogen intervention also delays bone loss in the vertebral bodies, both on computed tomography measurements and also on dual photon absorptiometry (Al-Azzawi et al, 1987). In our studies oestrogen-treated individuals had 29% more bone in their lumbar vertebrae after 10 years of therapy when compared with the placebo-treated population. Examination of lateral radiographs from these patients showed convincingly the presence of vertebral deformities in the placebo-treated group which were by and large absent from the oestrogen-treated individuals. If we assume that these deformations are the precursors of vertebral fracture, then it would appear that we are preventing about 75–80% of vertebral fractures with long-term use of oestrogens (Christiansen and Lindsay, 1991). Cross-sectional data from a Health Maintenance Organization confirms this conclusion (Ettinger et al, 1985). Here routine radiographs of postmenopausal women were reviewed and correlated with the use of oestrogen. Again vertebral deformations were significantly less obvious in the oestrogen-treated group. Epidemiological data are more difficult to obtain for vertebral fracture since these fractures may be asymptomatic and in any case rarely require hospital admission. Overall, however, the data support a dramatic reduction in the risk of vertebral fracture with long-term use of oestrogen.

Several of the epidemiological studies of hip fracture have also examined the effects of oestrogen on Colles' fracture and have shown a somewhat similar reduction in risk (Hutchinson et al, 1979; Weiss et al, 1980). This is perhaps not surprising since the majority of the data available on bone mass have made measurements in the radius, either at the usual mid-shaft site or more distally close to the site of fracture.

The majority of early studies involved only the use of oestrogen. More recently, however, the addition of a progestogen has been shown not to interfere with the dominant effects of oestrogen on the skeleton (Lindsay and Tohme, 1990). Certain progestogens, especially those derived from androgens, appear by themselves to reduce bone turnover and prevent bone loss (Abdalla et al, 1985). It is also possible that true progestogens can also prevent bone loss but in significantly greater doses than are usually used clinically (Gallagher et al, 1990).

Mechanism of action

The introduction of oestrogen therapy reverses the biochemical effects of the menopause or oophorectomy (Christiansen and Lindsay, 1991). There is generally found a small but significant reduction in serum calcium and phosphorous, accompanied by reduced urinary excretion of calcium and a fall in the tubular maximum for phosphate excretion. These latter changes suggest increased parathyroid hormone action on the kidney. Compatible with this is the apparent increase in urinary cyclic AMP excretion. Reduced bone turnover is suggested by a decline in serum alkaline phosphatase and oesteocalcin and by reduced urinary excretion of hydroxyproline and the cross-linking molecules of collagen deoxypyridinoline and pyridinoline.

Oestrogen prescription

Oestrogen therapy for postmenopausal women can be provided in one of several regimens. The common fashion is to give oestrogen on an intermittent basis, for 21 to 25 days of each calendar month. There is little logic to this regimen, however, unless to reduce breast tenderness, an occasional side-effect of oestrogens. Our practice is to give oestrogen daily and continuously. When given orally, we generally use conjugated equine oestrogen (Premarin) 0.625 mg per day or its equivalent. All oestrogens are effective in preventing bone loss, and thus preparations of oestrone or oestradiol can be substituted. There are also alternatives to the oral route, and oestrogens can be given transdermally (Estraderm, the 'oestrogen patch'), percutaneously as a cream or subcutaneously as a pellet with equal effects on the skeleton. Using the transdermal preparation requires continuous administration, since oestradiol levels fall quickly when the patch is removed, and if the patient has perimenopausal symptoms, these will return within a day or two.

For women who progress through menopause with their uterus in place, the addition of a progestin is required to protect the endometrium from the effects of exposure to long-term oestrogen. Oestrogen use in this population has been shown to increase the risk of endometrial hyperplasia and carcinoma from approximately 1:1000 to 2–10:1000 patient years (Cust et al, 1990). This effect is removed (reduced to baseline risk) when a progestin is added for 12–14 days per calendar month. The usual dose is medroxyprogesterone acetate 5–10 mg/day, beginning on the first day of each calendar month (Cust et al, 1990). This results in the return of menstrual bleeding for most patients and, although the bleeding is usually lighter than prior to the menopause, it seems unacceptable for some patients and many internists. With this regimen bleeding should occur between the eleventh and twenty-first day of the calendar month. Bleeding at other times requires investigation.

An alternative method for progestin provision is to give a lower dose of progestin (medroxyprogesterone acetate 2.5 mg) given continuously along with the oestrogen. For many patients this combination therapy causes endometrial hypoplasia and no bleeding. A significant proportion of patients will experience some light intermittent bleeding during the first 6 months of therapy, but this stops in most patients, although we do not usually use this combined continuous regimen in patients close to menopause, since they seem to have a higher incidence of more severe bleeding.

ADJUNCTS TO OESTROGEN THERAPY

Nutrition

It is still not clear if bone mass during the perimenopausal years can be influenced significantly by calcium intake (Heaney, 1991). While it is possible that a subset of the population will be calcium deficient and will lose skeletal mass as a consequence, it has proved extremely difficult to demonstrate this in prospective studies. It is unlikely that calcium could be expected to make up for the lack of oestrogen, and in fact the data tend to support this conclusion. A summary of the results indicates a small effect for calcium, occurring principally in peripheral cortical bone (Heaney, 1991). In part this is because the consequence of oestrogen withdrawal is an intrinsic alteration in skeletal metabolism. The addition of more calcium to the diet might, to some extent, offset the reduction in absorption efficiency that is a secondary effect of the increase in calcium efflux from the skeleton. However, because the changes in bone remodelling are intrinsic to the skeleton, this increased supply of calcium will simply result in increased loss of calcium in the urine and faeces. Replacement of calcium in bone would require that the extra supply of calcium reversed the changes that occur in the skeleton following oestrogen withdrawal at menopause.

Mostly, despite the mixed results of studies, it is generally considered reasonable to provide an intake of 1000–1500 mg/day to avoid any exacerbation of oestrogen deficiency by an inadequate calcium intake. This, it should be remembered, is total intake and supplements should only be provided where necessary to bring intake into that range. A simple and reasonably reliable (enough for general clinical use) assessment of calcium intake can be obtained by reviewing the intake of dairy produce, which for most adults provides 80% or more of the calcium intake. It is preferable to provide a nutrient from food sources, but because of the calories (and cholesterol) involved most women in this age group prefer to add calcium in tablet form. Usually a supplement of 500–600 mg/day is sufficient.

There does appear to be merit in providing adequate calcium intake for those presenting at an older age or with osteoporotic fractures (Dawson-Hughes et al, 1990; Heaney, 1991), since they have a clinical disorder that may be exacerbated by calcium deficiency. Since, as we have noted, the clinician does not have a readily available test for calcium deficiency, the response must be to ensure that all patients with clinical osteoporosis, at least, are given sufficient calcium to reduce the likelihood of increasing bone loss to maintain serum calcium within its tight limits. The mixed response of the clinical studies suggests perhaps that differing patient populations contain variable numbers of individuals who are actually calcium deficient. This could easily happen because of differing recruitment criteria, variable adaptation to low calcium intakes, or variation in the prevalence of other factors affecting the skeleton such as physical activity. Thus, in order to determine exactly the effect of calcium on the skeleton in calcium-deficiency osteoporosis a cohort of patients with true calcium deficiency would need to be identified. This study has yet to be designed and completed. In the absence of such data the recommendation that all at risk of osteoporosis receive sufficient calcium to ensure that none have an insufficient intake seems prudent.

Physical activity

The skeleton responds to physical stress in a somewhat analogous way to the response of skeletal muscle. Therefore, ensuring that the skeleton is adequately stressed seems appropriate. Since there is no specific exercise prescription for the skeleton, we generally follow guidelines for cardiovascular health and recommend 30 min of aerobic exercise three times per week. This should probably be accompanied by resistive exercises to strengthen the upper girdle and back. Patients over 35 years who have not participated in exercise previously should be evaluated by their physician before beginning a programme. Patients with osteoporosis should have their exercise programme supervised by a trained physiotherapist.

CONCLUSIONS

Bone loss after the menopause is a major cause of osteoporosis among women. This loss of skeletal tissue is a direct consequence of declining oestrogen secretion by the ovary. The specific intervention for prevention and treatment is oestrogen replacement, for which considerable data now exist confirming reduction in rate of bone loss at all ages in the postmenopausal population. Oestrogens should be given with a progestin when the uterus is still present. For osteoporosis, the decision to treat can be based on bone mass measurement. Other risk factors need to be evaluated at the same time, including nutritional and lifestyle factors, and altered where appropriate. Oestrogen therapy needs to be given for a long period and the benefits and potential risks need to be clearly explained to the patient.

Acknowledgements

This work was supported in part by PHS Grants AR39191 and DK42392.

REFERENCES

Abdalla HI, Hart DM, Lindsay R, Leggate I & Hooke A (1985) Prevention of bone loss in postmenopausal women by norethisterone. *Obstetrics and Gynecology* **6:** 789–792.

Aitken JM, Hart DM & Lindsay R (1973) Oestrogen replacement therapy for prevention of osteoporosis after oophorectomy. *British Medical Journal* **iii:** 515–518.

Al-Azzawi F, Hart DM & Lindsay R (1987) Long-term effect of oestrogen replacement therapy on bone mass as measured by dual photon absorptiometry. *British Medical Journal* **294:** 1261–1262.

Albright F (1947) The effect of hormones on osteogenesis in man. *Recent Progress in Hormone Research* **1:** 293–353.

Albright F, Bloomberg F & Smith PH (1940) Postmenopausal osteoporosis. *Transactions of the Association of American Physicians* **55:** 298–305.

Albright F, Smith PH & Richardson AM (1941) Postmenopausal osteoporosis. *Journal of the American Medical Association* **116:** 2465–2474.

Aloia JF, Cohn SH, Babu T, Abesamis C, Kalice N & Ellis K (1978) Skeletal mass and body composition in marathon runners. *Metabolism: Clinical and Experimental* **27:** 104–107.

Arnett TR, Lindsay R & Dempster DW (1986) Effect of estrogen and anti-estrogens on osteoclast activity in vitro. *Journal of Bone and Mineral Research* **1(supplement 1):** A99.

Bankson DD, Rifai N, Williams ME, Silverman LM & Gray TK (1989) Biochemical effects of 17β-estradiol on UMR106 cells. *Bone and Mineral* **6:** 55–63.

Burch JC, Byrd BF & Vaughn WK (1974) The effects of long-term estrogen on hysterectomized women. *American Journal of Obstetrics and Gynecology* **118:** 778–782.

Cann CE, Genant HK, Ettinger B et al (1980) Spinal mineral loss in oophorectomized women. *Journal of the American Medical Association* **244:** 2056–2059.

Christiansen C & Rodbro P (1983) Does postmenopausal bone loss respond to estrogen replacement therapy independent of bone loss rate. *Calcified Tissue International* **35:** 720–722.

Christiansen C & Rodbro P (1984) Does oestriol add to the beneficial effect of combined hormonal prophylaxis against early postmenopausal osteoporosis. *British Journal of Obstetrics and Gynaecology* **91:** 489–493.

Christiansen C & Lindsay R (1991) Estrogens, bone loss and preservation. *Osteoporosis International* **1:** 7–13.

Christiansen C, Christiansen MS & McNair P (1980) Prevention of early postmenopausal bone loss: conducted 2 years' study in 315 normal females. *European Journal of Clinical Investigation* **10:** 273–279.

Christiansen C, Christiansen MS & Transbol I (1981) Bone mass in postmenopausal women after withdrawal of estrogen/gestagen replacement therapy. *Lancet* **i:** 459–461.

Christiansen C, Riis BJ & Rodbro P (1987) Prediction of rapid bone loss in postmenopausal women. *Lancet* **i:** 1105–1107.

Christiansen C, Riis BJ & Rodbro P (1990) Screening procedure for women at risk of developing postmenopausal osteoporisis. *Osteoporosis International* **1:** 35–40.

Civitelli R, Agnusdei D, Nardi P, Zacchei F, Avioli LV & Gennari C (1988) Effects of one-year treatment with estrogens on bone mass, intestinal calcium absorption, and 25-hydroxy-vitamin D-1-hydroxylase reserve in postmenopausal osteoporosis. *Calcified Tissue International* **42:** 76–86.

Cummings SR, Black DM & Rubin SM (1989) Lifetime risks of hip, Colles', or vertebral fracture and coronary heart disease among white postmenopausal women. *Archives of Internal Medicine* **149:** 2445–2448.

Cust MP, Gangar KF & Whitehead MI (1990) Oestrogens and cancer. In Drive JO & Studd JWW (eds) *Hormone Replacement Therapy in Osteoporosis*, pp 177–195. London: Springer-Verlag.

Dawson-Hughes B, Dallal GE, Krall GE et al (1990) A controlled trial of the effect of calcium supplementation on bone density in postmenopausal women. *New England Journal of Medicine* **323:** 878–883.

Delmas P (1988) Biochemical markers of bone turnover. In Riggs BL & Melton LJ III (eds) *Osteoporosis: Etiology, Diagnosis and Management*, pp 297–316. New York: Raven Press.

Dempster DW, Shane E, Horbert W & Lindsay R (1986) A simple method for correlative light and scanning electron microscopy of human iliac crest bone biopsies: qualitative observations in normal and osteoporotic subjects. *Journal of Bone and Mineral Research* **1:** 15–21.

Draper HH (1985) Osteoporosis. *Advances in Nutritional Research* **7:** 172–186.

Eriksen EF, Colvard DS, Berg NJ et al (1988) Evidence of estrogen receptors in normal human osteoblast-like cells. *Science* **241**: 84–86.

Ernst M, Schmid CM & Foresch ER (1988) Enhanced osteoblast proliferation and collagen gene expression by estradiol. *Proceedings of the National Academy of Sciences of the USA* **85**: 2307–2310.

Ernst M, Heath JK & Rodan GA (1989) Estradiol effects on proliferation, messenger ribonucleic acid for collagen and insulin-like growth factor-I, and parathyroid hormone-stimulated adenylate cyclase activity in osteoblastic cells from calvariae and long bones. *Endocrinology* **125**: 825–833.

Ettinger B, Genant HK & Cann CE (1985) Long-term estrogen therapy prevents bone loss and fracture. *Annals of Internal Medicine* **102**: 319–324.

Ettinger B, Genant HK & Cann CE (1987) Postmenopausal bone loss is prevented by treatment with low-dosage estrogen with calcium. *Annals of Internal Medicine* **106**: 40–45.

Firooznia H, Golimbu C, Rafii M et al (1986) Rate of spinal trabecular bone loss in normal perimenopausal women: CT measurement. *Radiology* **161**: 735–738.

Fukayama S & Tashjian AH (1989) Direct modulation by estradiol of the response of human bone cells (SaOS-2) to human parathyroid hormone (PTH) and PTH-related protein. *Endocrinology* **124**: 397–401.

Gallagher JC, Kable WT & Goldgar D (1990) Effect of progestin therapy on cortical and trabecular bone: comparison with estrogen. *American Journal of Medicine* **90**: 171–178.

Gardsell P, Johnell O, Nilsson BE et al (1989) The predictive value of fracture, disease, and falling tendency for fragility fractures in women. *Calcified Tissue International* **45**: 327–330.

Garnett T, Savvas M & Studd JWW (1990) Reversal of bone loss with percutaneous oestrogens. In Drife JO & Studd JWW (eds) *HRT and Osteoporosis*, pp 295–314. London: Springer-Verlag.

Genant HK, Ettinger B, Harris ST, Block JE & Steiger P (1988) Quantitative computed tomography in assessment of osteoporosis. In Riggs BL & Melton LJ III (eds) *Osteoporosis: Etiology, Diagnosis and Management*, pp 221–249. New York: Raven Press.

Genant HK, Block JE, Steiger P et al (1989) Appropriate use of bone densitometry. *Radiology* **170**: 817–822.

Gowen M, Wood DD, Ihrie EJ, McGuire MKB & Russell RGG (1983) An interleukin-1-like factor stimulates bone resorption in vitro. *Nature* **306**: 378–380.

Gray TK, Flynn TC, Gray KM & Nabell LM (1987) 17β-Estradiol acts directly on the clonal osteoblastic cell line UMR106. *Proceedings of the National Academy of Sciences of the USA* **85**: 6267–6271.

Gray TK, Mohan S, Linkhart TA & Baylink DJ (1989) Estradiol stimulates in vitro the secretion of insulin-like growth factors by the clonal osteoblastic cell line, UMR 106. *Biochemical and Biophysical Research Communications* **158**: 407–412.

Heaney RP (1991) Calcium supplements: practical considerations. *Osteoporosis International* **1**: 65–71.

Heaney RP, Recker RR & Saville PD (1978a) Menopausal changes in calcium balance performance. *Journal of Laboratory and Clinical Medicine* **92**: 953–963.

Heaney RP, Recker RR & Saville PD (1978b) Menopausal changes in bone remodeling. *Journal of Laboratory and Clinical Medicine* **92**: 964–970.

Henneman PH & Wallach S (1957) A review of the prolonged use of estrogens and androgens in postmenopausal and senile osteoporosis. *Archives of Internal Medicine* **100**: 705–709.

Horsman A, Gallagher JC, Simpson M & Nordin BEC (1977) Prospective trial of estrogen and calcium in postmenopausal women. *British Medical Journal* **ii**: 789–792.

Hui SL, Slemenda CW & Johnston CC (1988) Age and bone mass as predictors of fracture in a prospective study. *Journal of Clinical Investigation* **81**: 1804–1809.

Hui SL, Slemenda CW & Johnston CC Jr (1990) The contribution of bone loss in postmenopausal osteoporosis. *Osteoporosis International* **1**: 30–34.

Hutchinson TA, Polansky SM & Feinstein AR (1979) Post-menopausal oestrogen protects against fractures of hip and distal radius. A case-control study. *Lancet* **ii**: 705–709.

Johnston CC, Melton LJ III, Lindsay R & Eddy DM (1989) Clinical indications for bone mass measurement. *Journal of Bone and Mineral Research* **4(supplement 2)**: 1–28.

Kiel DP, Felson DT, Anderson JJ, Wilson PWF & Moskowvitz MA (1987) Hip fracture and the use of estrogens in postmenopausal women. The Framingham study. *New England Journal of Medicine* **317**: 1169–1174.

Komm BS, Terpening CM & Benz DJ (1988) Estrogen binding, receptor mRNA, and biologic response in osteoblast-like osteosarcoma cells. *Science* **241:** 81–84.

Kreiger N, Kelsey JL, Holford TR & O'Connor T (1982) An epidemiologic study of hip fractures in postmenopausal women. *American Journal of Epidemiology* **116:** 141–148.

Lindsay R (1984) Osteoporosis and its relationship to estrogen. *Contemporary Obstetrics and Gynecology* **63:** 201–224.

Lindsay R (1988) Sex steroids in the pathogenesis and prevention of osteoporosis. In Riggs BL (ed.) *Osteoporisis: Etiology, Diagnosis and Management*, pp 333–358. New York: Raven Press.

Lindsay R & Tohme J (1990) Estrogen treatment of patients with established postmenopausal osteoporosis. *Obstetrics and Gynecology* **76:** 290–295.

Lindsay R, Aitken JM, Anderson JB, Hart DM, MacDonald EB & Clark AC (1976) Long-term prevention of postmenopausal osteoporosis by oestrogen. *Lancet* **i:** 1038–1041.

Lindsay R, Hart DM, MacLean A, Clark AC, Kraszewski A & Garwood J (1978a) Bone response to termination of oestrogen treatment. *Lancet* **i:** 1325–1327.

Lindsay R, Hart DM, Purdie P, Ferguson MM, Clark AC & Kraszewski A (1978b) Comparative effects of oestrogen and a progestogen on bone loss in postmenopausal women. *Clinical Science and Molecular Medicine* **54:** 193–195.

Lindsay R, Hart DM, Forrest C & Baird C (1980) Prevention of spinal osteoporosis in ooophorectomized women. *Lancet* **ii:** 1151–1154.

Lindsay R, Coutts JRT, Sweeney A & Hart DM (1984a) Endogenous oestrogen and bone loss following oophorectomy. *Calcified Tissue Research* **22:** 213–216.

Lindsay R, Hart DM & Clark DM (1984b) The minimum effective dose of estrogen for prevention of postmenopausal bone loss. *Obstetrics and Gynecology* **63:** 759–763.

Lindsay R, Mellish R, Cosman F & Dempster DW (1990) Biochemical markers of bone remodeling. In Nordin BEC (ed.) *Osteoporisis: Contributions to Modern Management*, pp 47–56. Lancashire, UK: Parthanon Publishing Group.

Lindsay R, Cosman F, Herrington BS & Himmelstein S (1991) Bone mass and body composition in normal women. *Journal of Bone and Mineral Research* **7:** 55–63.

Mazess RB & Mather W (1974) Bone mineral content of North Alaskan Eskimos. *American Journal of Clinical Nutrition* **27:** 916–925.

Mazess RB & Wahner HM (1988) Nuclear medicine in densitometry. In Riggs BL & Melton LJ III (eds) *Osteoporosis: Etiology, Diagnosis, and Management*, pp 251–295. New York: Raven Press.

Meema HE (1966) Menopausal and aging changes in muscle mass and bone mineral content. *Journal of Bone and Joint Surgery* **48A:** 1138–1144.

Meema S, Bunker ML & Meema HE (1975) Preventive effect of estrogen on postmenopausal bone loss. *Archives of Internal Medicine* **135:** 1436–1440.

Murrills R, Stein L & Dempster DW (1990) Contrasting effects of recombinant human interleukin-1 alpha and parathyroid hormone on isolated osteoclasts. *Calcified Tissue International* **46(supplement 2):** 43.

Nachtigall LE, Nachtigall RH & Nachtigall RD (1979) Estrogen replacement therapy I: a 10-year prospective study in the relationship to osteoporosis. *Obstetrics and Gynecology* **53:** 277.

Oursler M, Pyfferoen J, Osdoby P, Riggs B & Spelsberg T (1990) Osteoclasts express mRNA for estrogen receptor. *Journal of Bone and Mineral Research* **5(supplement 2):** 203.

Pacifici RL, Rifas L, Teitelbaum S et al (1987) Spontaneous release of interleukin 1 from human blood monocytes reflects bone formation in idiopathic osteoporosis. *Proceedings of the National Academy of Sciences of the USA* **84:** 4616–4620.

Pacifici R, Rifas L, McCracken R et al (1989) Ovarian steroid treatment blocks a postmenopausal increase in blood monocyte interleukin 1 release. *Proceedings of the National Academy of Sciences of the USA* **86:** 2398–2402.

Paganini-Hill A, Ross RK, Gerkins VR, Henderson BE, Arthur M & Mack TM (1981) Menopausal estrogen therapy and hip fractures. *Annals of Internal Medicine* **95:** 28–31.

Parfitt AM (1979) Quantum concept of bone remodeling and turnover implications for the pathogenesis of osteoporosis. *Calcified Tissue International* **28:** 1–5.

Parfitt AM (1988) Bone remodeling: relationship to the amount and structure of bone, and the pathogenesis and prevention of fractures. In Riggs BL & Melton LJ III (eds) *Osteoporosis: Etiology, Diagnosis, and Management*, pp 45–94. New York: Raven Press.

Peacock M & Selby P (1986) The effect of transdermal oestrogen on bone, calcium regulating hormones and liver in postmenopausal women. *Clinical Endocrinology* **25**: 543–547.

Price PA, Parthemore JG & Deftos LJ (1980) New chemical marker for bone metabolism. Measurement by radioimmunoassay of bone GLA protein in the plasma of normal subjects and patients with bone disease. *Journal of Clinical Investigation* **66**: 878–883.

Riggs BL & Melton LJ III (1986) Involutional osteoporosis. *New England Journal of Medicine* **314**: 1676–1686.

Riggs BL, Jowsey J, Kelly PJ, Jones JD & Maher FT (1969) Effect of sex hormones on bone in primary osteoporosis. *Journal of Clinical Investigation* **48**: 1065–1072.

Riggs BL, Wahner HW, Dunn WL, Mazess RB, Offord KP & Melton LJ III (1981) Differential changes in bone mineral density of the appendicular and axial skeleton with aging: relationship to spinal osteoporosis. *Journal of Clinical Investigation* **67**: 328–335.

Riis B, Thomsen K, Strom V & Christiansen C (1987) The effect of percutaneous estradiol and natural progesterone on postmenopausal bone loss. *American Journal of Obstetrics and Gynecology* **156**: 61–65.

Ross PD, Wasnich RD & Vogel JM (1988) Detection of prefracture spinal osteoporosis using bone mineral absorptiometry. *Journal of Bone and Mineral Research* **3**: 1–11.

Schmid C, Ernst M, Zapf J & Foresch ER (1989) Release of insulin-like growth factor carrier proteins by osteoblasts: stimulation by estradiol and growth hormone. *Biochemical and Biophysical Research Communications* **160**: 788–794.

Slemenda C, Hui SL, Longcope C & Johnston CC (1987a) Sex steroids and bone mass: a study of changes about the time of the menopause. *Journal of Clinical Investigation* **80**: 1261–1269.

Slemenda CW, Hui SL, Johnston CC Jr & Longcope C (1987b) Prediction of bone mass and rate of loss: clinical versus laboratory data. *Journal of Bone and Mineral Research* **2**: 206.

Slemenda CW, Hui SL, Longcope C, Wellman H & Johnston CC Jr (1990) Predictors of bone mass in perimenopausal women: a prospective study of clinical data using photon absorptiometry. *Annals of Internal Medicine* **112**: 96–101,

Steiniche T, Hasling C, Charles P et al (1989) A randomized study of the effects of estrogen/gestagen or high dose oral calcium on trabecular bone remodeling in postmenopausal osteoporosis. *Bone* **10**: 313–320.

Stevenson JC, Lees B, Devenport M, Cust MP & Ganger KF (1989) Determinants of bone density in normal women: risk factors for future osteoporosis? *British Medical Journal* **298**: 924–928.

Stevenson JC, Cust MP, Gangar KF, Hillard TC, Lees B & Whitehead MI (1990) Effects of transdermal versus oral hormone replacement therapy on bone density in spine and proximal femur in postmenopausal women. *Lancet* **336**: 265–269.

Van Hemert AM, Vandenbroucke JP, Birkenhager JC & Valkenburg HA (1990) Prediction of osteoporotic fractures in the general population by a fracture risk score. *American Journal of Epidemiology* **132**: 123–135.

Weiss NS, Ure CL & Ballard JH (1980) Decreased risk of fractures of the hip and lower forearm with postmenopausal use of oestrogen. *New England Journal of Medicine* **303**: 1195–1198.

6

Hormone replacement therapy for established osteoporosis in elderly women

CLAUS CHRISTIANSEN

It is now established that postmenopausal oestrogen therapy stops further bone loss (Lindsay et al, 1976; Christiansen et al, 1981) and, if started in due time and continued long enough, decreases the number of osteoporotic fractures (Weiss et al, 1980; Ettinger et al, 1985). A number of studies have furthermore shown that oestrogens in combination with different pro-gestogens have the same effect on early postmenopausal bone loss as un-opposed oestrogen therapy (Riis et al, 1987a,b).

Treatment of symptomatic postmenopausal osteoporosis still remains a problem. Whereas the 85-year-old woman with severe osteoporosis is generally acknowledged to be out of therapeutic reach, the treatment of the 65-year-old woman showing the first signs of osteoporosis would certainly be worthwhile, if this was possible. In an earlier study we demonstrated that treatment with 17β-oestradiol (17βE$_2$) in sequential combination with norethisterone acetate (norethindrone acetate *USP*; NETA) induced a continuous increase in bone mineral content (BMC) in 70-year-old women (Jensen et al, 1982). These results have been confirmed by a recent study with the same oestrogen/progestogen regimen, which also produced an increased BMC in early postmenopausal women (Munk-Jensen et al, 1988).

Our first study was followed up by an investigation of the effect of continuous combined 17βE$_2$ and NETA in elderly women with osteoporosis (Christiansen and Riis, 1990). This treatment regimen is compared in a way which should prevent any endometrial bleeding.

Figure 1 shows the individual changes in BMC occurring over 1 year of treatment (per cent values) with either 2 mg 17βE$_2$ + 1 mg NETA + 500 mg of calcium (Sandoz)® ($n = 20$) or a placebo combined with the same calcium supplementation ($n = 20$). At four measurement sites, the mean BMC was increased in the hormone group as compared with the placebo group ($P < 0.05$). Bone mass in the ultradistal forearm and in the spine showed a difference between the hormone and the placebo group of about 8%, whereas the differences in the distal forearm and in the total skeleton were about 3% and 5%, respectively.

Figure 2 shows the mean percentage changes in the four bone compartments over 2 years of treatment. The women receiving the active treatment had an increased bone mass of 3.6–13.1%, out of the 28 individual

Baillière's Clinical Obstetrics and Gynaecology—
Vol. 5, No. 4, December 1991
ISBN 0–7020–1548–2

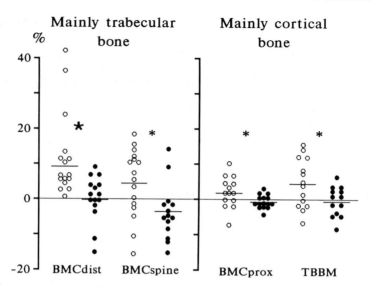

Figure 1. Individual changes in bone mass measurements after 1 year of treatment with $17\beta E_2 + NETA$ (○) or placebo (●). dist = ultradistal forearm; prox = distal forearm. From Christiansen and Riis (1990), with permission.

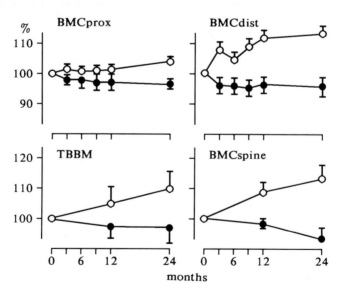

Figure 2. Mean changes in bone mass measurements over 2 years of treatment with $17\beta E_2 + NETA$ (○) or placebo (●). Abbreviations as for Figure 1. From Christiansen and Riis (1990), with permission.

changes in the hormone group only one was below zero, whereas 34 out of the 40 values in the control group were negative.

A large number of clinical studies have been performed in recent years in order to find a therapeutic agent able to increase bone mass in osteoporotic subjects. The study populations have often comprised relatively old post-menopausal women with spinal crush fractures and thus a severe degree of osteoporosis. Women with a moderate degree of osteoporosis with a BMC averaging 25% below that of premenopausal women may be a more realistic target group for treatment.

Oestrogen is known to depress bone turnover, primarily by decreasing bone resorption. Owing to the coupling of the resorption and formation processes, bone formation will also be depressed after some time of oestrogen treatment (Parfitt, 1984). Postmenopausal women treated for a couple of months with oestrogen monotherapy will thus achieve a steady state in bone turnover similar to that in premenopausal women. The result is a cessation of bone loss and a future constant bone mass. Treatment with $17\beta E_2$ and NETA, however, increased bone mass significantly. The increase we observed in bone mineral may be transient and may reach a maximum level when a new steady state in bone remodelling has occurred. The increase in bone mass was more pronounced in the sites of the skeleton with a rather high content of trabecular bone (distal forearm, spine) than in those with a high content of cortical bone (proximal forearm, total skeleton), i.e. the treatment seems to be more effective in trabecular bone.

The concept of a 'fracture threshold' is still somewhat unclear, but it is often believed that when 20% of the bone mass has been lost the fracture risk increases seriously. If bone mass could be measured at a point where the loss was not too severe, for instance when a forearm fracture occurs, a couple of years on $17\beta E_2 + $ NETA treatment could produce a timely and important increase in bone mass, even if the increase levels off after a couple of years. As the new bone is normal in structure and histology (Pødenphant et al, 1988), this would probably mean a substantial decrease in the risk of fracture.

Other groups have studied the effect of hormone replacement therapy in elderly women with osteoporosis. Quigley et al (1987) studied 397 post-menopausal women and found that even users over the age of 65 showed continued protection from bone loss as long as therapy was continued (Quigley et al, 1987). In a recent study from the Mayo Clinic it was further-more demonstrated that oestrogen replacement therapy reduced fracture incidence in osteoporotic women (Lufkin et al, 1990). Hormone replacement therapy is therefore also a realistic alternative for the treatment of established osteoporosis, as stated at the last Consensus Development Conference (1991) on osteoporosis.

REFERENCES

Christiansen C, Christensen MS & Transbøl I (1981) Bone mass in postmenopausal women after withdrawal of oestrogen/gestagen replacement therapy. *Lancet* i: 459–461.

Christiansen C & Riis BJ (1990) 17β-estradiol and continuous norethisterone: a unique treatment for established osteoporosis in elderly women. *Journal of Clinical Endocrinology and Metabolism* **71:** 836–841.

Consensus Development Conference (1991) Prophylaxis and treatment of osteoporosis. *American Journal of Medicine* **90:** 107–110.

Ettinger B, Genant HK & Cann CE (1985) Long-term estrogen replacement prevents bone loss and fractures. *Annals of Internal Medicine* **102:** 319–324.

Jensen GF, Christiansen C & Transbøl I (1982) Treatment of postmenopausal osteoporosis. A controlled therapeutic trial comparing oestrogen/gestagen, 1,25-dihydroxyvitamin D3 and calcium. *Clinical Endocrinology* **16:** 515–524.

Lindsay R, Aitken JM, Anderson JB, Hart DM, MacDonald EB & Clarke AC (1976) Long-term prevention of postmenopausal osteoporosis by oestrogen. *Lancet* **i:** 1038–1040.

Lufkin EG, Hodgson SF, Kotowicz MA, O'Fallon WM, Wahner HW & Riggs BL (1990) The use of transdermal estrogen treatment in osteoporosis. In Christiansen C & Overgaard K (eds) *Osteoporosis 1990.* Proceedings of the Third International Symposium on Osteoporosis, Copenhagen, Denmark, 14–20 October, vol. 3, pp 1995–1998. Osteopress.

Munk-Jensen N, Nielsen SP, Obel EB & Eriksen PB (1988) Reversal of postmenopausal vertebral bone loss by oestrogen and progestogen: a double blind placebo controlled study. *British Medical Journal* **296:** 1150–1152.

Parfitt AM (1984) The cellular basis of bone remodeling: the quantum concept reexamined in light of recent advances in the cell biology of bone. *Calcified Tissue International* **36:** 37–45.

Pødenphant J, Riis BJ, Johansen JS, Leth A & Christiansen C (1988) Ilia crest biopsy in longitudinal therapeutic trials of osteoporosis. *Bone and Mineral* **5:** 77–87.

Quigley MED, Pervis PL, Burnin AM & Brooks P (1987) Estrogen therapy arrests bone loss in elderly women. *American Journal of Obstetrics and Gynecology* **156:** 1516–1523.

Riis BJ, Jensen J & Christiansen C (1987a) Cyproterone acetate, an alternative gestagen in postmenopausal oestrogen/gestagen therapy. *Clinical Endocrinology* **26:** 327–334.

Riis BJ, Thomsen K, Strøm V & Christiansen C (1987b) The effect of percutaneous estradiol and natural progesterone on postmenopausal bone loss. *American Journal of Obstetrics and Gynecology* **156:** 61–65.

Weiss NS, Carol PH, Ure CL et al (1980) Decreased risk of fractures of the hip and lower forearm with postmenopausal use of estrogen. *New England Journal of Medicine* **303:** 1195–1198.

7

Do we have any alternative to sex steroids in the prevention and treatment of osteoporosis?

CHARLES H. CHESNUT III

Oestrogen hormone therapy is a potent and beneficial therapy for both preventing and treating osteoporosis; it is also of value for relieving post-menopausal symptoms and for positively affecting cardiovascular disease. However, not all women can, or wish to, utilize oestrogen replacement therapy; are there alternative therapies? The answer is yes, as there are now available an increasing number of alternatives to oestrogen, either approved for usage by regulatory authorities in various countries or under development.

BASIC PRINCIPLES OF THE THERAPY OF OSTEOPOROSIS

Consideration of alternative therapies (to sex steroids) for osteoporosis must involve some consideration of bone remodelling and the effects on this of various treatments. Osteoporosis, particularly the postmenopausal variety, may be thought of as an abnormality of bone remodelling at the tissue level, and various therapies are aimed at correcting such bone remodelling abnormalities.

Bone is constantly turning over, as the skeleton responds to the biomechanical effects of loading and as it functions as a reservoir for calcium. As noted in Figure 1, the first event in normal remodelling is an increase in bone resorption mediated by the osteoclast; this is followed within a period of perhaps 45 to 70 days by increased bone formation directed by the osteoblast. These two processes are, perhaps homeostatically, coupled, such that with normal bone remodelling there is no net change in the amount of bone mass present (an initial increase or decrease in bone resorption is followed by a corresponding increase or decrease in bone formation). As noted in part (c) of Figure 1, in osteoporosis there is most frequently an increase in bone resorption over normal levels, leading to an increased bone mass loss; bone formation does not 'couple' normally to the increase in bone resorption, and an incremental loss of bone mass takes place. In addition, some individuals developing osteoporosis (particularly those treated with corticosteroids) may have as their primary problem a decrease in bone formation (panel (d) of Figure 1); the end result is the

Baillière's Clinical Obstetrics and Gynaecology—
Vol. 5, No. 4, December 1991
ISBN 0–7020–1548–2

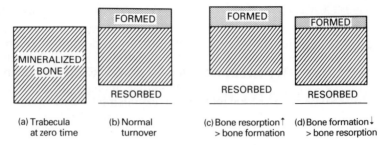

Figure 1. Osteoporosis due to disruption of normal bone remodelling sequences. (a) and (b) denote a bony trabecula at zero time and normal bone turnover, respectively. (c) and (d) denote two possible mechanisms of abnormal bone remodelling. From Chesnut & Kribbs (1982).

same, with a net loss in bone mass. Since bone mass is the principal determinant of fracture, such a loss of bone mass is associated with an increased risk for fractures. Based upon these principles, the ideal therapy for osteoporosis would be one which inhibits bone resorption (and prevents further bone loss) and stimulates formation (and replaces bone mass previously lost). Currently no therapy, including oestrogen replacement therapy, is available that can accomplish both of these particular actions; there are, however, a number of therapies, alternatives to oestrogen, that can perform one or other of these actions, i.e. a decrease in bone resorption or a stimulation of bone formation.

As noted in Table 1, a number of therapies are available to inhibit bone resorption and prevent loss, including calcium, oestrogen, synthetic salmon calcitonin, the bisphosphonates and vitamin D compounds (which secondarily decrease bone resorption by increasing calcium absorption in the gut). A number of agents are available to stimulate bone formation, including sodium fluoride, anabolic steroids, amino acid fragments of the intact parathyroid hormone, the vitamin D congener calcitriol, and exercise. These alternative therapeutic agents will be discussed in detail.

Table 1. Therapies for osteoporosis.

Inhibitors of bone resorption
Calcium
Oestrogen
Calcitonin
Bisphosphonates
Vitamin D (secondarily, by increasing calcium absorption)
Stimulators of bone formation
Anabolic steroids/testosterone
Sodium fluoride
Intact parathyroid hormone fragments
Growth factors
Calcitriol
Exercise

It should be noted that the majority of clinical trials assessing these osteoporosis therapies over the past 20 years have utilized bone mass (most typically at the spine and wrist) as the primary end-point of treatment efficacy, rather than prevention of fracture. Such bone mass end-points are necessary due to the large and frequently unavailable patient numbers required for studies evaluating a therapy's effect upon fractures; such end-points, however, are reasonable as an exponential relationship exists between decreasing bone mass and increasing fracture risk (Ross et al, 1988; Slemenda et al, 1990). Presumably a stabilization or improvement in bone mass is associated with a lesser risk for fracture. In addition, the majority of therapies discussed are used for the preservation of bone mass and by extrapolation for the prevention of fractures; with the exception of synthetic salmon calcitonin, the majority of the medications discussed have little immediate effect upon the acute pain syndrome associated with osteoporosis and its fractures.

THERAPEUTIC AGENTS INHIBITING BONE RESORPTION

Calcium

A therapeutic rationale exists for the usage of oral calcium in the prevention and treatment of osteoporosis, in that increased calcium intake hypothetically results in a slight increase in serum calcium, and a consequent decrease in parathyroid hormone-mediated bone resorption. Such changes, may, however, be transient, and may not occur in every individual. Studies have shown that calcium deficiency exists in many females (Consumer Nutrition Center, 1980) and that increased calcium intake may be of value in individuals who are calcium deficient (Burnell et al, 1986; Dawson-Hughes et al, 1990); however, identifying those individuals with calcium deficiency is difficult. There are few longitudinal double-blind controlled studies documenting a beneficial effect of calcium on bone mass and fracture reduction; a number of cross-sectional and epidemiological studies, however, do suggest such an effect (Matkovic et al, 1979; Holbrook et al, 1988). Nevertheless, an adequate calcium intake is mandatory for individuals at risk for, or with, osteoporosis; increased calcium intake in the absence of hyperparathyroidism or kidney stones is associated with few side-effects (occasional bloating and constipation), is relatively inexpensive, and is logistically simple to acccomplish from either dietary or calcium supplement sources. An intake of 1000 to 1500 mg of elemental calcium per day may be recommended for women, particularly adolescent females (Matkovic et al, 1990; Miller and Johnston, 1990), pregnant females and elderly females with osteoporosis—the elderly control subjects in three recently completed clinical trials did not lose bone mass at multiple skeletal sites over periods of 2 to 4 years, and received only increased calcium intake (Ott and Chesnut, 1989; Riggs et al, 1990; Watts et al, 1990). Calcium is, however, not a surrogate for oestrogen in women immediately after the menopause (Riis et al, 1987). Sources of calcium may be milk and dairy products or calcium supplements; if supplements are utilized, calcium carbonate provides the greatest percentage of elemental calcium. Calcium citrate and calcium phosphate are also reasonable calcium supplements. The bioavailability of any utilized calcium supplement should be assured.

Adequate calcium intake is a mainstay of any programme for preventing or treating osteoporosis.

Calcitonin

The therapeutic rationale for the usage of calcitonin in osteoporosis includes its ability to inhibit osteoclastic activity and osteoclast recruitment and to thereby decrease bone resorption. Synthetic salmon calcitonin is the preparation usually utilized, although human and eel calcitonins are also available. Synthetic salmon calcitonin has been shown to stabilize bone mass over a period of 2 to 3 years in the total skeleton (Gruber et al, 1984) and in the spine and hip (Civitelli et al, 1988) in osteoporotic female populations; it has not been proven to prevent fractures, but such an effect would appear reasonable, given the hypothesis that stabilization of bone mass is associated with a lesser fracture risk. Also, calcitonin may be more effective in individuals with high bone remodelling (increased bone turnover) (Civitelli et al, 1988). Calcitonin is currently administered by either parenteral injection or through a nasal spray (Reginster et al, 1987; Overgaard et al, 1990) for both prevention and treatment of osteoporotic disease. A dosage of 50 to 100 units daily administered either subcutaneously or intramuscularly is indicated for established disease; due to a potential downregulation of receptor sites, however, a dosage of 50 to 100 units every second or third day may be more efficacious over time. If the nasal spray route of administration is utilized, a dosage of 200 to 400 units daily will be of value for either individuals with osteoporosis or for its prevention. Lastly, calcitonin possesses an analgesic effect, quite separate from its bone sparing effect; such an effect is presumably mediated by stimulation of β-endorphin secretion. Usage of synthetic salmon calcitonin, usually parenterally, at a dosage of 100 units nightly for perhaps 1 to 2 weeks may be of value in the individual with a recent acute compression fracture (Pun and Chan, 1989).

As noted, synthetic salmon calcitonin is a valuable treatment for the stabilization of bone mass in the osteoporotic female patient. In addition, increasing evidence supports the usage of synthetic salmon calcitonin administered by nasal spray as a prophylactic treatment for individuals at risk for osteoporosis. In this light it can be thought of as an alternative to oestrogen replacement therapy; one study does show a similar effect of human calcitonin to oestrogen in the stabilization of bone mass in women soon after the menopause (MacIntyre et al, 1988).

Calcitonin, either salmon or eel, is approved for osteoporosis therapy in many countries throughout the world.

Bisphosphonates

A therapeutic rationale for the bisphosphonates (etidronate, alendronate, tiludronate, clodronate, etc.) exists in that these agents 'chemisorb' to bone crystal and thereby presumably prevent access of the osteoclast (and of its resorbing activity) to bone crystal. In addition, there is presumably a direct effect of bisphosphonates in reducing the number and activity of osteoclasts. Data currently available (Storm et al, 1990; Watts et al, 1990) from studies utilizing the bisphosphonate etidronate, at a dosage of 400 mg daily administered intermittently 2 weeks out of every 3 months on an empty stomach, indicate a stabilization of spinal bone mass, and a prevention of spinal fractures, in a female osteoporotic population followed over 2 (Watts et al, 1990) to 3 (Storm et al, 1990) years. With the exception of mild diarrhoea, no side-effects of this medication were noted. In this light it should be noted that, as a class, bisphosphonates do reduce bone remodelling; hypothetically, such a reduction in bone remodelling over a prolonged period of time may impede the healing of microfractures. Such a hypothesis is unproven, however; on-going studies do not show any such adverse effects over 4 years. It should however be noted that etidronate, if administered continuously rather than intermittently, may produce a mineralization defect in bone.

The bisphosphonates, specifically etidronate, have approval in a number of countries in Europe and Asia for usage in the treatment or prevention of osteoporosis. Undoubtedly in the future one or another of these bisphosphonates will be utilized as a major therapeutic modality in osteoporosis, and in this sense this class of compounds possesses perhaps the greatest potential for usage as alternatives to oestrogen replacement therapy.

Vitamin D metabolites

The therapeutic rationale for the usage of vitamin D and its metabolites in osteoporosis consists primarily of the action of vitamin D in stimulating the production of calcium binding protein at the gut level, and thereby increasing calcium absorption. In addition, the in vitro actions of active metabolites of vitamin D such as calcitriol (1,25-dihydroxycholecalciferol) include a stimulation of bone formation (Stern, 1980). However, no more than 1000 units of vitamin D_2 are needed to assure adequate calcium in the elderly or osteoporotic patient, and a multiple vitamin with 150 to 400 iu of D_2 per day may be quite adequate (Dawson-Hughes et al, 1991; Meunier et al, 1991). A high intake of vitamin D (perhaps greater than 1000 units per day), in the absence of cortisone usage, is potentially deleterious; vitamin D administered in suprapharmacological dosages may be associated with hypercalciuria (and an increased risk for kidney stones and nephrocalcinosis), hypercalcaemia, and a worsening of osteoporosis (presumably through a permissive effect of vitamin D in high dosage on parathyroid hormone-mediated bone resorption) (Chesnut, 1992).

Whether congeners of vitamin D such as 1,25-dihydroxycholecalciferol are of primary value in the treatment of osteoporosis remains unclear (Tilyard et al, 1992); while there may be a beneficial effect of calcitriol in osteoporosis, it would appear from current studies (Ott and Chesnut, 1989) that the dosage necessary to achieve a beneficial effect on bone mass and fractures is too high to avoid renal toxicity.

It should be noted that, while a multiple vitamin with small amounts of vitamin D may be viewed as adjunctive therapy for the prevention and treatment of osteoporosis and may be of value along with oestrogen in preventing this disease, vitamin D and its congeners cannot be viewed as an alternative to oestrogen replacement therapy, at least at this time. However, on-going clinical trials with newer vitamin D congeners shown to have a smaller calcaemic and calciuric effect may indeed prove of value in osteoporosis.

Vitamin D congeners are prescribed most frequently in Asiatic countries; given the diminished calcium intake in these countries, such usage in minimal dosage may be appropriate, at least to increase calcium absorption at the gut level.

TREATMENTS FOR OSTEOPOROSIS WHICH STIMULATE BONE-FORMATION

Sodium fluoride

The therapeutic rationale for the usage of sodium fluoride in osteoporosis, primarily for treating established disease, depends on fluoride's ability to stimulate the osteoblast to make new bone. When fluoride is administered, however, the bone produced will be composed of fluorapatite crystal instead of hydroxyapatite crystal. Studies (Riggs et al, 1990) demonstrate an improvement in spinal bone mass when fluoride is administered in dosages of 65 to 75 mg of sodium fluoride per day; however, no decrease in the number of spine fractures, and an increase in non-spine fractures (including the hip), has been noted in the study group receiving fluoride (compared with the placebo control group). The concern with sodium fluoride is that, although bone mass quantity may indeed increase when sodium fluoride is administered, the quality of the bone formed may be suspect (possibly due to the presence of fluorapatite crystal), with an increased, rather than decreased, risk for fracture. Other studies (Mamelle et al, 1988) have suggested benefit from fluoride; however, on balance the questions regarding the structural integrity of bone formed with fluoride, coupled with its side-effects (gastric upset and possible gastric ulceration, an increase in arthritic symptoms, a possible increase in stress fractures and a syndrome of plantar fasciitis) probably prohibit its widespread usage. Whether lower dosages of sodium fluoride or differing preparations (such as the sustained release capsule) will be associated with skeletal benefit and fewer side-effects is unproven at present.

Sodium fluoride cannot therefore be viewed as an alternative to oestrogen replacement therapy at this time. While it is available and utilized in a number of areas throughout the world, close supervision and monitoring of patients receiving this medication is imperative.

Anabolic steroids

The therapeutic rationale for the anabolic steroids (i.e. stanozolol, nandrolone decanoate) in the treatment of osteoporosis consists of their ability, similar to sodium fluoride, to stimulate the osteoblast to form new bone. Bone mass is seen to increase when these agents are administered (Chesnut et al, 1983; Need et al, 1989). However, the side-effects of anabolic steroids include masculinization in women, potential liver toxicity and a negative effect on lipids (Taggart et al, 1982) (possibly predisposing to an increased risk of cardiovascular disease); these side-effects, and their abuse in young athletes, have led to restriction on the use of these agents in the United States.

Anabolic steroids, therefore, may occasionally be of value in the individual patient not responding to other forms of therapy for osteoporosis, but cannot be viewed as alternatives to oestrogen replacement therapy. They should never be used for the prevention of osteoporosis, and any administration of these medications should be with full cognizance on the part of both physician and patient of their potential for side-effects.

Exercise

A therapeutic rationale for the usage of exercise in the prevention and treatment of osteoporosis may be made on the basis of the hypothetical increase in bone remodelling leading to an increase in bone formation over bone resorption, and a net accrual of bone mass. The type of exercise (weight bearing?), the duration of exercise, the effect of detraining, etc. remain unclear; stringent controlled studies in osteoporosis are lacking to document a beneficial effect of exercise in increasing or stabilizing bone mass and preventing fractures. While exercise cannot be a surrogate for oestrogen in the prevention of bone loss immediately after the menopause (Prince et al, 1991), as with calcium it does however seem reasonable to recommend an exercise programme for the individual at risk for, or with, oesteoporosis; inactivity and disuse are obviously deleterious to the skeleton, presumably by negatively influencing remodelling with an increase in resorption over formation.

The future for therapeutic agents stimulating bone formation

Although effective and safe bone-forming agents are currently lacking, the future for this area of osteoporosis therapy is bright. A number of additional therapeutic agents which stimulate bone formation are currently under development, including anabolic fragments of parathyroid hormone (amino acid fragments of the hormone which may paradoxically stimulate bone formation, rather than stimulate bone resorption as would be anticipated when the intact parathyroid hormone molecule is administered). Also, growth factors such as transforming growth factor β and insulin-like growth factors I and II are under investigation. These agents would primarily be utilized in treating established disease (replacing bone mass previously lost) rather than in prevention, although if such agents are safe, inexpensive and easily administered, they would probably have a potential prophylactic value as well.

CONCLUSIONS

In conclusion, there are a number of alternatives (particularly calcitonin and the bisphosphonates) to oestrogen replacement therapy in the prevention and treatment of osteoporosis. The majority of these therapies are presumably as equally effective as oestrogen in preserving bone mass and possibly in preventing fractures (etidronate). However, it should be noted that oestrogen replacement therapy has a number of potential beneficial effects in addition to its skeletal actions; with the exception of the analgesic effect of calcitonin, the alternative therapies discussed act primarily upon the skeleton, with little beneficial effect for other organ systems.

REFERENCES

Burnell JM, Baylink DJ, Chesnut CH III & Teubner EJ (1986) The role of skeletal calcium deficiency in postmenopausal osteoporosis. *Calcified Tissue International* **38:** 187–192.

Chesnut CH III (1992) Osteoporosis and its treatment. *New England Journal of Medicine* **326:** 406–408 (editorial).

Chesnut CH & Kribbs PJ (1982) Osteoporosis: some aspects of pathophysiology and therapy. *Journal of Prosthetic Dentistry* **48:** 4.

Chesnut CH III, Ivey JL, Gruber HE et al (1983) Stanozolol in postmenopausal osteoporosis: therapeutic efficacy and possible mechanisms of action. *Metabolism: Clinical and Experimental* **32:** 571–580.

Civitelli R, Gonelli S, Zacchei F et al (1988) Bone turnover in postmenopausal osteoporosis. *Journal of Clinical Investigation* **83:** 1268–1274.

Consumer Nutrition Center (1980) *Food and Nutrient Intakes of Individuals in One Day in the United States, Spring, 1977. Nationwide Food Consumption Survey 1977–78, Preliminary Report No. 2.* Hyattsville, Maryland: United States Department of Agriculture.

Dawson-Hughes B, Dallal GE, Krall EA et al (1990) A controlled trial of the effect of calcium supplementation on bone density in postmenopausal women. *New England Journal of Medicine* **323:** 878–883.

Dawson-Hughes B, Dallal GE, Krall EA et al (1991) Effect of vitamin D supplementation on wintertime and overall bone loss in healthy postmenopausal women. *Annals of Internal Medicine* **115:** 505–512.

Gruber H, Ivey J, Baylink D et al (1984) Long-term calcitonin therapy in postmenopausal osteoporosis. *Metabolism: Clinical and Experimental* **33:** 295–303.

Holbrook TL, Barrett-Connor E & Wingard DL (1988) Dietary calcium and risk of hip fracture: fourteen-year prospective population study. *Lancet* **ii:** 1046–1049.

MacIntyre I, Whitehead M, Banks L et al (1988) Calcitonin for prevention of postmenopausal bone loss. *Lancet* **i:** 900–902.

Mamelle N, Meunier PJ, Dusan R et al (1988) Risk-benefit ratio of sodium fluoride treatment in primary vertebral osteoporosis. *Lancet* **ii:** 361–365.

Matkovic V, Kostia LK, Simonovic I et al (1979) Bone status and fracture rates in two regions of Yugoslavia. *American Journal of Clinical Nutrition* **50:** 1244–1259.

Matkovic V, Fontana D, Tominac C, Goel P & Chesnut CH III (1990) Factors that influence peak bone mass formation: a study of calcium balance and the inheritance of bone mass in adolescent females. *American Journal of Clinical Nutrition* **52:** 878–888.

Meunier PJ, Chapuy MC, Arlot ME et al (1991) Effects of a calcium and vitamin D₃ supplement on non-vertebral fracture rate, femoral bone density and parathyroid function in elderly women. A prospective placebo-controlled study. *Journal of Bone and Mineral Research* **6(supplement 1):** 210, S135 (abstract).

Miller JZ & Johnston CC (1990) Relationship of dietary calcium and bone mass in twin children. *Journal of Bone and Mineral Research* **5(supplement 2):** 275 (abstract 805).

Need AG, Horowitz M, Bridges A et al (1989) Effects of nandrolone decanoate and antiresorptive therapy on vertebral density in osteoporotic postmenopausal women. *Archives of Internal Medicine* **149:** 57–60.

Ott SM & Chesnut CH III (1989) Calcitriol treatment is not effective in postmenopausal osteoporosis. *Annals of Internal Medicine* **110:** 267–274.

Overgaard K, Hansen MA, Nielsen VAH et al (1990) Discontinuous calcitonin treatment of established osteoporosis: effects of withdrawal of treatment. *American Journal of Medicine* **89:** 1–6.

Prince RL, Smith M, Dick IM et al (1991) Prevention of postmenopausal osteoporosis. A comparative study of exercise, calcium supplementation, and hormone-replacement therapy. *New England Journal of Medicine* **325:** 1189–1195.

Pun KK & Chan LWL (1989) The analgesic effect of intranasal salmon calcitonin in the treatment of osteoporotic vertebral fractures. *Clinical Therapeutics* **11(2):** 87–89.

Reginster J, Albert A, Lecarte M et al (1987) 1-Year controlled randomized trial of prevention of early postmenopausal bone loss by intranasal calcitonin. *Lancet* **ii:** 1481–1483.

Riggs BL, Hodgson SF, O'Fallon WM et al (1990) Effect of fluoride treatment on the fracture rate in postmenopausal women with osteoporosis. *New England Journal of Medicine* **322:** 802–809.

Riis B, Thomsen K & Christiansen C (1987) Does calcium supplementation prevent postmenopausal bone loss? A double-blind, controlled clinical study. *New England Journal of Medicine* **316:** 173–177.

Ross PD, Wasnich RD & Vogel JM (1988) Detection of pre-fracture spinal osteoporosis using bone mineral absorptiometry. *Journal of Bone and Mineral Research* **3:** 1–11.

Slemenda CW, Hui SL, Longcope C, Wellman H & Johnston CC Jr (1990) Predictors of bone mass in perimenopausal women, a prospective study of clinical data using photon absorptiometry. *Annals of Internal Medicine* **112:** 96–101.

Stern PH (1980) The D vitamins and bone. *Pharmacological Reviews* **32:** 47–80.

Storm T, Thamsborg G, Steiniche T et al (1990) Effect of intermittent cyclical etidronate therapy on bone mass and fracture rate in women with postmenopausal osteoporosis. *New England Journal of Medicine* **322:** 1265–1271.

Taggart HA, Applebaum-Bowden D, Haffner S et al (1982) Reduction in high density lipoproteins by anabolic steroid (stanozolol) therapy for postmenopausal osteoporosis. *Metabolism: Clinical and Experimental* **3:** 1147–1152.

Tilyard MW, Spears GFS, Thomson J et al (1992) Treatment of postmenopausal osteoporosis with calcitriol or calcium. *New England Journal of Medicine* **326:** 357–362.

Watts NB, Harris ST, Genant HK et al (1990) Intermittent cyclical etidronate treatment of postmenopausal osteoporosis. *New England Journal of Medicine* **323:** 73–79.

8

Effects of sex steroids on serum lipids and lipoproteins

JYTTE JENSEN

Coronary heart disease (CHD) is the major cause of death in both men and women in Western countries, accounting for about one-third of all deaths in both sexes. Despite the similar dimension of this major health problem in the sexes, gender differences exist in the time of manifestation of this arteriosclerotic endpoint.

Prior to the menopause, the incidence of CHD is substantially lower in women than in men, whereas once past the menopause the incidence of CHD in women increases and approaches that of men. The relative protection of young and middle-aged women has generally been attributed to the impact of female sex hormones.

Since epidemiological studies have established that serum lipids and lipoproteins are important determinants of CHD in both men and women, and sex hormones are known to be potent lipid-altering agents, the possibility has been advanced that the female mortality advantage might be mediated through an influence of sex steroids on lipid metabolism. As a consequence, attention has been focused on the lipid metabolic effects of endogenous female sex hormones, especially in relation to the menopause, and the potential cardioprotective actions of postmenopausal hormone replacement therapy—which is increasingly used for alleviation of climacteric symptoms, urogenital atrophy and prevention of postmenopausal bone loss—have received substantial interest.

SERUM LIPIDS AND LIPOPROTEINS

Lipoproteins are spherical particles that serve as transport vehicles for lipids in plasma. Four major lipoproteins fractions are classified according to their density by preparative ultracentrifugation: chylomicrons, very low density lipoproteins (VLDL), low density lipoproteins (LDL) and high density lipoproteins (HDL). Chylomicrons and VLDL, the largest lipoproteins, consist mainly of triglycerides which are transported to extrahepatic tissues and/or act as energy sources. The VLDL particle is converted to LDL by intravascular hydrolysation of the triglycerides catalysed by the lipoprotein lipase (LPL).

Baillière's Clinical Obstetrics and Gynaecology—
Vol. 5, No. 4, December 1991
ISBN 0–7020–1548–2

LDL is the major carrier of cholesterol, conveying up to 70% of the plasma cholesterol, which is transported to peripheral tissues. Removal of LDL from plasma is mainly mediated by the LDL-receptor, which recognizes the apolipoprotein B; however, non-specific pathways, the so-called 'scavenger pathway', also seem to be present. HDL comprise a heterogeneous group of particles, but is generally subdivided into two fractions: the larger HDL_2, which is rich in lipids, and the more dense protein-rich particle HDL_3. HDL_3 receives cholesterol from peripheral cells, which is esterified by lecithin-cholesterol acyltransferase (LCAT) producing HDL_2, and in turn transported back to the liver for degradation.

Determinants of lipids and lipoproteins

Lipid and lipoprotein metabolism is complex and is influenced by numerous factors, including sex, heredity, diet, obesity, exercise, alcohol consumption, smoking habits, socioeconomic status and a variety of drugs (Bush et al, 1988). These factors may have direct or indirect influence on lipid metabolism and their actions may be independent and synergistic.

Age and sex are important determinants of lipids and lipoproteins. Serum total cholesterol, LDL cholesterol (LDL-C) and VLDL cholesterol (VLDL-C) as well as triglycerides increase with age in both sexes, but levels are significantly higher in men than in women throughout the age range of 20 to 50 years (Heiss et al, 1980; Connor et al, 1982). Around the age of 50 years, a cross-over occurs in the sex-related lipid and lipoprotein pattern, resulting in higher serum total cholesterol and LDL-C concentrations in women throughout the older ages, whereas serum triglycerides and VLDL-C concentrations in women approach those observed in men. HDL cholesterol (HDL-C) concentrations remain, by contrast, significantly higher in women than in men throughout adult life.

LIPIDS, LIPOPROTEINS AND CARDIOVASCULAR DISEASE

Epidemiological studies have established that serum total cholesterol and LDL-C are important predictors of morbidity and mortality from CHD (Kannel et al, 1971; Gordon et al, 1977a; Martin et al, 1986). In addition, a strong inverse and independent relationship has been demonstrated between HDL-C and the risk of CHD (Miller et al, 1977; Castelli et al, 1986), whereas the discriminant power of the separate HDL subfractions have not yet been established (Miller, 1987). CHD is the major clinical sign of progressive atherosclerosis, and evidence that lipoproteins play an important role in the pathogenesis of atherosclerosis is substantial. The clinical significance of the observed relationship between lipoproteins and CHD has been further strengthened by intervention trials examining the effect of altering lipids and lipoproteins on the risk of CHD. Several intervention studies have demonstrated that the risk of CHD can be reduced by reducing serum total cholesterol and LDL-C levels. The joint results of dietary and drug intervention trials have demonstrated that for each 1% reduction achieved in serum cholesterol, the risk of CHD is reduced by 1.5–2% (Tyroler, 1987). Increases in HDL-C have been reported to be associated with an additional reduction in CHD risk (Lipid Research Clinics Program, 1984). Unfortunately, most studies, including intervention studies, have been performed in men, and despite the fact that lipids and lipoproteins are established as important determinants of CHD in women also (Castelli et al, 1986), no comparative evidence exists on the preventive effect of lipid modification in women.

The role of triglycerides as a predictor of cardiovascular disease is controversial. Serum triglycerides do not appear to be an independent risk factor for CHD in men (Hulley et al, 1980), but have been suggested to be a strong predictor of CHD in women over 50 years of age (Kannel et al, 1971; Lapidus et al, 1985b). Although the relationship in women might be explained by a concurrent association with diabetes (Gordon et al, 1977b), the exact influence of triglycerides on the risk of CHD remains to be clarified.

THE MENOPAUSE AND SERUM LIPIDS AND LIPOPROTEINS

The role of the menopause as an independent risk factor for cardiovascular disease remain controversial. Several studies have reported an increased risk of atherosclerosis and cardiovascular disease after the occurrence of natural or surgical menopause (Bengtsson and Lindquist, 1978; Gordon et al, 1978; Rosenberg et al, 1981; Witteman et al, 1989). The Framingham study examined 1598 women, and found an overall relative risk of CHD in postmenopausal women of 2.7 (Gordon et al, 1978). No differences were observed in the risk of CHD between women with a natural menopause and those with a surgical menopause. Rosenberg et al (1981) reported a relative risk of non-fatal myocardial infarction of 2.9 in young oophorectomized women compared with age-matched premenopausal women. The relative risk of CHD increased with decreasing age at menopause, a finding which was also reported by others (Bengtsson and Lindquist, 1978; Gordon et al, 1978). Colditz et al (1987) found an increased risk of CHD (relative risk of 2.2) only in oophorectomized women, whereas natural menopause had no apparent influence. Other studies have reported no association between menopause and the risk of cardiovascular disease (Manchester et al, 1971; Blanc et al, 1977; Lapidus et al, 1985a).

Attempts to clarify the effect of the menopause on standard cardiovascular risk factors have revealed little evidence of menopause-related alterations in body weight, hypertension, smoking habits or glucose intolerance (Hjortland et al, 1976; Lindquist and Bengtsson, 1980; Kannel and Gordon, 1987) which might explain the increased risk. The only marked influence of the menopause appears to be a change in lipid and lipoprotein profiles. Cross-sectional studies have almost consistently reported higher concentrations of serum total cholesterol and triglycerides in postmenopausal women compared with age-matched premenopausal women (Kannel and Gordon, 1987; Lindquist and Bengtsson, 1980; Bush et al, 1984; Bonithon-Kopp et al, 1990), and these findings have been confirmed in longitudinal studies (Lindquist, 1982; Matthews et al, 1989; Egeland et al, 1990; Jensen et al, 1990). The increments have been observed following both natural and surgical-induced menopause.

Studies on individual lipoproteins have shown that the menopausal rise in total cholesterol is confined to LDL-C (Bush et al, 1984; Matthews et al, 1989; Bonithon-Kopp et al, 1990; Farish et al, 1990; Jensen et al, 1990), whereas data on HDL-C have been conflicting. HDL-C has been reported to be unaffected by changes in ovarian function in cross-sectional studies (Bush et al, 1984; Bonithon-Kopp et al, 1990) and in one prospective study (Farish et al, 1990); however, three recent prospective studies have concurrently reported small, but significant decreases in HDL-C following the menopause (Matthews et al, 1989; Egeland et al, 1990; Jensen et al, 1990).

The lipid metabolic effects of the natural menopause are shown in Figure 1. Serum total cholesterol and LDL-C concentrations increase by 5–7% and 10–12%, respectively, and serum triglycerides increase by 8–10%, whereas HDL-C levels are reduced by approximately 4–6%. Apart from the changes in HDL-C, menopausal alterations in lipids and lipoproteins have been shown to occur within 3–6 months after the cessation of menstrual bleedings (Jensen et al, 1990), and the simultaneously occurring decreases in serum oestrogens concomitant with significant increases in serum gonadotrophins reflect a close relation to the ceased ovarian function (Jensen et al, 1990). In contrast, changes in HDL-C may occur gradually throughout the peri- and postmenopausal years (Jensen et al, 1990).

Epidemiological studies have shown that serum total cholesterol and LDL-C increase as a function of biological age (Heiss et al, 1980; Lindquist and Bengtsson, 1980; Connor et al, 1982). Age, however, seems merely a partial explanation for premenopausal changes in lipids and lipoproteins. In

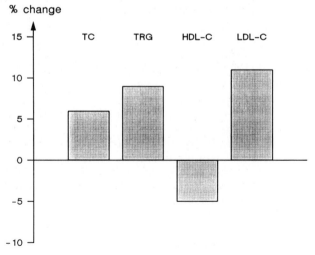

Figure 1. Menopausal changes in serum lipids and lipoproteins observed in longitudinal studies. TC = total cholesterol; TRG = triglycerides.

a cross-sectional study from Göteborg (Lindquist and Bengtsson, 1980), increases in serum total cholesterol were related to the remaining premenopausal time. In accordance, Matthews et al (1989) reported significantly higher baseline levels of serum total cholesterol and LDL-C in the women who were to experience their menopause within the following 2½ years compared with their premenopausal controls. Jensen et al (1990) observed increases in total cholesterol and LDL-C when subdividing perimenopausal women approaching the menopause according to the degree of menstrual irregularity. These findings suggest that, in addition to the abrupt increase observed at the time of cessation of ovarian hormone production, serum total cholesterol and LDL-C increase gradually during the years preceding the menopause, and might be a consequence of deteriorating ovarian function.

Whether the postmenopausal increments in total cholesterol and LDL-C observed in both cross-sectional and longitudinal studies (Heiss et al, 1980; Lindquist and Bengtsson, 1980; Connor et al, 1982; Lindquist, 1982; Jensen et al, 1990) are a function of biological age or occur as a consequence of advancing postmenopausal age cannot be answered directly because of interdependency between the two. However, Lindquist and Bengtsson (1980) observed increases in total cholesterol with increasing postmenopausal age, and associations between serum lipids and biological age in postmenopausal women have been insignificant (Klorfajn et al, 1978; Jensen et al, 1990).

In summary, serum lipids and lipoproteins are significantly altered as a consequence of the menopause, resulting in more atherogenic lipid profiles in the postmenopausal years. The menopausal changes probably explain the cross-over pattern in lipid and lipoprotein profiles observed between the sexes around the age of 50 years (Heiss et al, 1980; Connor et al, 1982) and might in part be responsible for the increased cardiovascular risk observed in postmenopausal women.

OESTROGEN MONOTHERAPY AND SERUM LIPIDS AND LIPOPROTEINS

Oral oestrogens

Numerous studies have almost consistently shown that treatment with oral exogenous oestrogens in postmenopausal women reduces the serum total cholesterol and LDL-C, whereas HDL-C increases, particularly the HDL_2 fraction (reviewed by Bush and Miller, 1987; Rijpkema et al, 1990). These changes, which correlate with a reduced risk of CHD in epidemiological studies, have been shown in both normal and hyperlipidaemic women, and in women with natural and surgical menopause. Various formulations, including synthetic oestrogens (i.e. ethinyloestradiol, mestranol), conjugated equine oestrogens and natural (human) oestrogens (17β-oestradiol, oestradiol valerate), have been shown to elicit similar qualitative effects on LDL-C and HDL-C, whereas their effects on serum triglycerides differ.

Synthetic formulations invariably increase serum triglycerides, which is also a prevalent finding with conjugated equine oestrogens, whereas data on 'natural' oestrogens have been conflicting (Bush and Miller, 1987).

Changes in lipids and lipoproteins are dose-related (Jensen et al, 1987a; Bush and Miller, 1987; Krauss et al, 1988), but even with similar doses, the reported changes have been quite wide, probably owing to differences in laboratory methods, small study populations—often comprising a mix of young and old menopausal women—dissimilar treatment durations, and lack of controls. Bush and Miller (1987) adjusted the changes reported in various studies for sample size and treatment duration. Overall, natural oestrogens had the most favourable effects on lipids and lipoproteins, with reductions in serum total cholesterol and LDL-C of 4% and 16%, respectively, and increases in HDL-C and triglycerides of 15% and 4% following a conventional dose of oestradiol valerate (2 mg/day). Conjugated equine oestrogens (0.625 mg and 1.25 mg) were found to produce less pronounced changes, except on serum triglycerides, which were increased by 20%, whereas synthetic oestrogens induced changes two to three times greater than those observed following natural and conjugated oestrogens, resulting in marked increments in serum triglycerides (31%).

The underlying mechanisms for the lipid-modifying actions of oestrogens have not been established, but the triglyceride-elevating actions of synthetic oestrogens appear to be caused by increased production in the liver (Kissebah et al, 1973). Lowering of LDL-C might result from increased LDL-receptor synthesis as observed in animal studies (Kovanen et al, 1979), whereas increases in HDL-C may be the joint result of increased apolipoprotein A synthesis (Schaefer et al, 1983) and suppressed degradation of HDL particles due to inhibition of hepatic lipoprotein lipase (Tikkanen et al, 1986).

Non-oral routes of oestrogen administration

Postmenopausal oestrogen therapy is traditionally administrated by the oral route. However, enhanced induction of hepatic functions by oral oestrogen administration, probably owing to the very high concentrations of oestradiol and oestrone in liver sinusoids, might be linked to the potential side-effects of oestrogens. By parenteral administration of oestrogens, the first-pass effect of the liver is initially bypassed and the steroid-induced actions on the liver are minimized (Holst et al, 1983).

Non-oral routes of oestrogen administration have been proved clinically effective in postmenopausal hormone replacement therapy, but variable effects on lipids and lipoproteins have been reported.

Vaginal administration

Vaginal administration of conjugated oestrogens with increasing dosage (0.3 mg–2.5 mg) produced no changes in lipids and lipoproteins after 4 months of observation (Mandel et al, 1983), whereas significant increases in serum triglycerides and HDL-C and significant decreases in LDL-C were reported 24 days after vaginal administration of the potent ethinyloestradiol (50 μg/day) (Goebelsmann et al, 1985). The latter changes were comparable to those observed following oral administration of 10 μg ethinyloestradiol. Vaginal administration of a lower dose (20 μg) exerted similar trends, although changes were not significant.

Subcutaneous and intramuscular administration

In a 6-month study by Farish et al (1984), subcutaneous implants of 50 mg 17β-oestradiol resulted in significant reductions in serum total cholesterol (5%) and LDL-C (6%), and significant increases in HDL-C (7%) 4 months after implant insertion. However, in a later long-term study from the same group (Fletcher et al, 1986), no significant differences were observed between the menopausal women receiving oestrogen implants compared with untreated controls. Unfortunately, changes in relation to pretreatment values were not reported. Stanczyk et al (1988), using a similar implant, observed significant increases in HDL-C and no change in LDL-C during 6 months of observation. Sharf et al (1985) used a higher dose of pellets (100 mg), and reported a significant decrease in LDL-C of 23% and a significant increase in HDL-C of 32% 14 weeks after implantation. No significant changes in serum triglycerides and VLDL-C were reported following oestrogen implants.

Sherwin et al (1987) examined short-term changes in lipids and lipoproteins following intramuscular injection of 10 mg oestradiol valerate and observed a transient, but significant decrease in total cholesterol and LDL-C simultaneous with peak hormone values, whereas HDL-C continued to increase throughout the 28 days of the study.

Percutaneous and transdermal administration

Data on the actions of percutaneous oestrogens on lipid metabolism have been inconsistent. Basdevant et al (1983) reported significant reductions in serum total triglycerides and VLDL triglycerides after 2 months of treatment with percutaneous oestrogens (3 mg), and a similar although not significant reduction was reported by Elkik et al (1982) after 3 weeks of treatment. Serum total cholesterol, LDL-C and HDL-C remained unchanged in both studies. Fåhreaus et al (1982, 1983) reported a decreasing trend in serum total cholesterol and LDL-C following 6 months of percutaneous oestrogen therapy (3 mg), whereas no changes were observed in serum HDL-C and triglycerides. In a long-term placebo-controlled study, Jensen et al (1987c) reported significant reductions in total cholesterol and LDL-C concentrations of 4% and 8%, respectively, after 6 months of treatment, which were maintained throughout the 2 years of study. Serum concentrations of HDL-C and triglycerides increased slightly during therapy, and average responses were significantly increased compared with placebo after 1 year.

Transdermal oestrogen administration using patches containing doses of 25, 50, 100 and 200 μg oestradiol had no influence on serum lipids and lipoproteins in a short-term study (28 days) by Chetkowski et al (1986), although serum oestradiol concentrations comparable to the mid-follicular phase of premenopausal women were achieved by these doses. However, preliminary results of recent long-term studies of transdermal oestrogen administration (Adami et al, 1990; Lindgren et al, 1990) suggest that significant reductions are achieved in serum total cholesterol and LDL-C in the long run, whereas changes in serum HDL-C and triglycerides are small and insignificant.

In summary, parenteral administration of oestrogens apparently elicits qualitatively similar actions on serum lipids and lipoproteins as observed with oral administration. The parenteral route, however, modifies the lipid metabolic response, probably as a consequence of the avoidance of the first-pass liver effect. The reduced oestrogen load in the liver and the protracted steady-state seem to explain the quantitative differences as well as the delayed response compared with oral administration of oestrogens.

COMBINED OESTROGEN-PROGESTOGEN THERAPY

Addition of a progestogen to postmenopausal oestrogen therapy has become essential in women with an intact uterus (Consensus Report, 1988), since it has been shown to protect the endometrium from oestrogenic hyperstimulation and apparently eliminates the potential risk of oestrogen-induced endometrial cancer (Hammond et al, 1979; Gambrell et al, 1983; Persson et al, 1986).

Two principal types of synthetic progestogens are commonly employed in clinical practice in addition to 'natural' progesterone. The 19-nortestosterone derivatives include the 13-methyl-gonanes norethisterone acetate (NETA; norethindrone acetate *USP*), lynoestrenol, norethynodrel, and the 13-ethyl-gonanes DL-norgestrel (NORG), levonorgestrel (LNG), desogestrel (DG), norgestimate and gestodene. The 19-nortestosterone derivatives are characterized by the exhibition of some androgenic activities in addition to their progestational actions. The other principal type of synthetic progestogens, the 17-hydroxyprogesterone derivatives, which include medroxyprogesterone acetate (MPA), cyproterone acetate (CPA), megestrol acetate (MGA) and dydrogesterone (DD), have virtually no androgenic activities, and may even possess some antiandrogenic properties. Due to structural differences, however, progestogens within both main groups may cover a wide range of biological activities and relative potencies.

Progestogens may elicit changes in serum lipids and lipoproteins which are opposite to those observed with oestrogens, and qualitative differences seem to exist between the 19-nortestosterone and the 17-hydroxyprogesterone derivatives in this respect. Data on the effects of different combinations of oestrogen-progestogen therapy on lipid metabolism are summarized in

Tables 1 and 2, and for most studies concerned, results express the combined oestrogen-progestogen phase of the tablet cycle.

19-Nortestosterone derivatives

Negation or even reversal of the oestrogen-induced rise in serum HDL-C has generally been shown to be most pronounced following the addition of 19-nortestosterone-derived progestogens (Hirvonen et al, 1981, 1987; Ottosson et al, 1985), and these adverse actions have been attributed to the androgenic properties of the progestogen. 19-Nortestosterone derivatives may also counteract the oestrogen-induced reductions in LDL-C (Hirvonen et al, 1987), although this is controversial (Jensen et al, 1989), whereas their triglyceride-reducing capacity seem favourable. However, not only the qualitative differences between the 19-nortestosterone and the 17-hydroxyprogesterone derivatives, but also factors such as the dose and the relative biological activity are important determinants for the ultimate effect on serum lipids. This was clearly demonstrated in one of the first and most cited clinical trials on the effect of combined oestrogen-progestogen treatment, where Hirvonen et al (1981) reported significant reductions in HDL-C to 20% below baseline values following the addition of NETA (10 mg) and NORG (0.5 mg) to 2 mg oestradiol valerate in postmenopausal women. In comparison, no significant changes were observed with the addition of MPA (10 mg). Corresponding findings observed in other studies using high pharmacological doses of 19-nortestosterone derivatives (Silver-stolpe et al, 1982a,b) led to the general opinion that progestogens with androgenic properties were inappropriate for postmenopausal hormone replacement therapy due to their adverse effects on lipid metabolism. However, later studies have shown that the doses compared were highly unequipotent and—with respect to the 19-nortestosterone derivatives—much in excess of those required for adequate protection of the endometrium.

Adequate protection of the endometrium can be achieved by the addition of 1 mg NETA or 0.15 mg NORG (equivalent to 0.075 mg LNG) for 10 days each oestrogen cycle (Whitehead et al, 1981; Siddle et al, 1982; Whitehead, 1986) and studies employing these clinical relevant doses of progestogens have reported only minor alterations in the oestrogen-mediated changes in serum lipids and lipoproteins. Jensen et al (1986) examined the cyclic changes in serum lipids and lipoproteins during treatment with three different doses of 17β-oestradiol (1, 2, and 4 mg) combined with 1 mg NETA (for 10 days). Serum total cholesterol and LDL-C declined significantly in relation to the oestrogen dose and were not affected by the addition of NETA. The oestrogen-induced rise in HDL-C, on the other hand, was partly negated by the addition of NETA, but remained significantly higher than baseline values in the two higher oestrogen dose groups (2 mg and 4 mg). Concordant findings of significant reductions in serum total cholesterol and LDL-C and no significant changes in HDL-C have been reported in long-term studies using cyclic administration of minimum effective doses of NETA (1 mg), NORG (0.15 mg), LNG (0.075 mg) and DG (150 μg)

Table 1. Effects on lipid metabolism of different oestrogen-progestogen combinations including 19-nortestosterone derivatives in postmenopausal women.

Reference	Duration (months)	No.	Oestrogen/progestogen dose	% change			
				TC	TRG	HDL-C	LDL-C
DL-Norgestrel (NORG)							
Hirvonen et al, 1981	3	6	EV 2 mg + NORG 0.5 mg cy	−18*		−25*	
Hirvonen et al, 1990	12	18	EV 2 mg + NORG 0.5 mg cy	−17*	−20*	−23*	−14*
Farish et al, 1986	6	21	CE 0.625 mg + NORG 0.15 mg cy	−10*	−2	−5	−13*
Fletcher et al, 1987	12	11	CE 0.625 mg + NORG 0.15 mg cy	−10*	+7	−7	−11*
Levonorgestrel (LNG)							
Hirvonen et al, 1987	6	11	EV 2 mg + LNG 0.25 mg cy	−5	−31	−20***	+4
Hirvonen et al, 1987	6	11	EV 2 mg + LNG 0.25 mg cy	−13	−18	−19***	−1
Ottosson et al, 1985	3	20	EV 2 mg + LNG 0.25 mg cy	−3		−18**	
Lagrelius et al, 1986	12	42	EV 2 mg + LNG 0.25 mg cy	−4	−2***	−9***	
Lagrelius et al, 1986	12	43	EV 2 mg + LNG 0.125 mg cy	−6	−4	−1	
Haarbo et al, 1991	3	23	EV 2 mg + LNG 0.075 mg cy	−7**		−1	−11***
Marslew et al, 1991b	24	19	EV 2 mg + LNG 0.075 mg cy	−10***		−3	−15***

Norethisterone acetate (NETA)

Study			Oestrogen	Progestogen				
Hirvonen et al, 1981	3	6	EV 2 mg	+ NETA 10 mg cy	-12*		-20*	+30**
Silverstolpe et al, 1982b	1½	11	EV 2 mg	+ NETA 10 mg cy	+7	0	-31**	-19***
Jensen et al, 1986	2	10	E_2 4 mg + E_3	+ NETA 1 mg cy	-7**		+13*	-17***
Jensen and Christiansen, 1987	12	19	E_2 4 mg + E_3	+ NETA 1 mg cy[1]	-11***	+11	+15**	-15***
Jensen et al, 1986	2	10	E_2 2 mg + E_3	+ NETA 1 mg cy[1]	-4		+10*	-15***
Jensen and Christiansen, 1987	12	22	E_2 2 mg + E_3	+ NETA 1 mg cy	-6*	+1	+8	-8**
Jensen et al, 1986	2	10	E_2 1 mg + E_3	+ NETA 1 mg cy[1]	-4*		+2	-11*
Jensen and Christiansen, 1987	12	23	E_2 1 mg + E_3	+ NETA 1 mg cy	-4	-1	+15*	-8**
Mattsson et al, 1984	12	26	E_2 2 mg + E_3	+ NETA 1 mg co	-10*	-1	-20*	-8
Farish et al, 1989	12	38	E_2 2 mg	+ NETA 1 mg co	-2	-3	-7*	+1
Jensen et al, 1989	24	21	E_2 2 mg	+ NETA 1 mg co	-15***	+2	-7	-20***
Sporrong et al, 1989	12	15	E_2 2 mg	+ NETA 1 mg co	-14***	-3	-16**	-15**
Sporrong et al, 1989	12	15	E_2 2 mg	+ NETA 0.5 mg co	-16***	-6	-13	+4

Desogestrel (DG)

Study			Oestrogen	Progestogen				
Haarbo et al, 1991	3	24	E_2 1.5 mg	+ DG 0.15 mg cy	-6***		+2	-11**
Marslew et al, 1991a	24	20	E_2 1.5 mg	+ DG 0.15 mg cy	-8*		-1	-16***

TC = total cholesterol; TRG = triglycerides; EV = oestradiol valerate; CE = conjugated equine oestrogens; E_2 = 17β-oestradiol; E_3 = oestriol; cy = cyclic; co = continuous.

* $P < 0.05$.
** $P < 0.01$.
*** $P < 0.001$.
[1] Average during tablet cycle.

Table 2. Effects on lipid metabolism of different oestrogen-progestogen combinations including 17-hydroxyprogesterone derivatives or progesterone in postmenopausal women.

Reference	Duration (months)	No.	Oestrogen/progestogen dose	% change			
				TC	TRG	HDL-C	LDL-C
Medroxyprogesterone acetate (MPA)							
Hirvonen et al, 1981	3	6	EV 2 mg + MPA 10 mg cy	−8*		−7	
Hirvonen et al, 1987	6	11	EV 2 mg + MPA 10 mg cy	−2	−17	+7	−5
Hirvonen et al, 1987	6	11	EV 2 mg + MPA 10 mg cy	−7	−10	+5	−10
Ottosson et al, 1985	3	20	EV 2 mg + MPA 10 mg cy	−2		−8**	
Haarbo et al, 1991	3	23	EV 2 mg + MPA 10 mg cy	−9***		+4	−14***
Marslew et al, 1991a	24	18	EV 2 mg + MPA 10 mg cy	−9***		+2	−20***
Notelovitz et al, 1982	18	10	CE 0.625 mg + MPA 10 mg cy	−2	+30	+10	−16
Hargrove et al, 1989	12	5	CE 0.625 mg + MPA 10 mg cy	+3		+26**	
Prough et al, 1987	9	10	CE 0.625 mg + MPA 10 mg cy	0	−13	+25	−11
Notelovitz et al, 1982	18	10	CE 1.25 mg + MPA 10 mg cy	+9	+9	+18	−16
Weinstein, 1987	12	12	CE 0.625 mg + MPA 5 mg cy	−8*	+28	+11	−18*
Sherwin and Gelfand, 1989	12	25	CE 0.625 mg + MPA 5 mg cy	−2	+40**	+5	−4
Sherwin and Gelfand, 1989	12	20	CE 1.25 mg + MPA 5 mg cy	0	+43**	+14*	−9**
Weinstein, 1987	12	12	CE 0.625 mg + MPA 5 mg co	−7	+11	+3	−19
Weinstein, 1987	12	12	CE 0.625 mg + MPA 2.5 mg co	−10*	+32	+4	−21*
Prough et al, 1987	9	16	CE 0.625 mg + MPA 2.5 mg co	+1	+4	+13	+1

Cyproterone acetate (CPA)								
Jensen et al, 1989	24	32	EV 2 mg	+ CPA 1 mg cy	−5*	+8	+2	−8**
Hirvonen et al, 1990	12	18	EV 2 mg	+ CPA 1 mg cy	−24*	−13	−6	−18*
Haarbo et al, 1991	3	24	EV 2 mg	+ CPA 1 mg co	−5*		+3	−6*
Marslew et al, 1991b	24	19	EV 2 mg	+ CPA 1 mg co	−5*		+1	−10**
Megestrol acetate (MGA)								
Sporrong et al, 1989	12	15	E$_2$ 2 mg	+ MGA 2.5 mg co	−5	+25*	−10	−5
Sporrong et al, 1989	12	15	E$_2$ 2 mg	+ MGA 5 mg co	−14**	+3	−1	−22**
Dydrogesterone (DD)								
Fletcher et al, 1987	6	6	CE 0.625 mg	+ DD 10 mg cy	−3	−10	−2	0
Progesterone (PROG)								
Fåhreaus et al, 1983	6	11	E$_2$ percut 3 mg	+ PROG 300 mg cy	−1	+8	−14*	+4
Ottosson et al, 1985	3	18	EV 2 mg	+ PROG 200 mg cy	+1		0	−12***
Jensen et al, 1987c	12	20	E$_2$ percut 3 mg	+ PROG 200 mg cy	−7**		+5	
Hargrove et al, 1989	12	10	E$_2$ 0.7–1.1 mg	+ PROG 200–300 mg co	−11		+53	

TC = total cholesterol; TRG = triglycerides; EV = oestradiol valerate; CE = conjugated equine oestrogens; E$_2$ = 17β-oestradiol; percut = percutaneous; cy = cyclic; co = continuous.

* $P < 0.05$.
** $P < 0.01$.
*** $P < 0.001$.

added to conventional doses of oestrogens (Farish et al, 1986; Fletcher et al, 1987; Jensen and Christiansen, 1987; Haarbo et al, 1991; Marslew et al, 1991a,b), whereas higher progestogen doses invariably result in significant reductions in HDL-C (Lagrelius et al, 1986; Hirvonen et al, 1987, 1990). It should be noted that the dose of DG sufficient for endometrial protection in postmenopausal women has not yet been established in clinical trials, but was merely extrapolated from clinical experience with contraceptives.

From current data, it is evident that the dose of progestogen is of decisive importance for the ultimate effects on lipid metabolism of combined oestrogen-progestogen therapy, especially when 19-nortestosterone derivatives are considered, owing to their potential adverse actions. Cyclic treatment using minimum effective doses of 19-nortestosterone derivatives for endometrial protection can be accomplished without adverse actions on serum lipids and lipoproteins. Despite the cyclic abolishment of the oestrogenic actions on HDL-C, the favourable effects of oestrogens have been shown to be largely preserved (Jensen et al, 1986; Haarbo et al, 1991).

Continuous oestrogen-progestogen therapy reduces the frequency of withdrawal bleedings (Staland, 1981; Mattsson et al, 1982; Jensen et al, 1987b) and may consequently increase patient compliance. Expanding the time of progestogen administration, however, may eventually lead to an imbalance in the oestrogenic and progestogenic actions on lipid metabolism. Oestrogen-induced reductions in total cholesterol and LDL-C do not appear to be affected in continuous oestrogen-progestogen therapy (Jensen et al, 1987b, 1989; Sporrong et al, 1989), but may actually be enhanced. However, most studies using continuous combinations with 19-nortestosterone derivatives have reported reductions in HDL-C (Mattson et al, 1984; Farish et al, 1989; Jensen et al, 1989; Sporrong et al, 1989) and, although reductions were not statistically significant in all studies, a suppressive action seems evident. Whether the dose of progestogen during continuous administration, on the other hand, can be further reduced without loss of endometrial protection remains to be established.

17-Hydroxyprogesterone derivatives and natural progesterone

The 17-hydroxyprogesterone derivatives have generally been considered relatively inert with respect to lipid metabolism. Early studies on the effect of the addition of MPA reported no interference with lipoprotein metabolism (Hirvonen et al, 1981; Notelovitz et al, 1982; Silverstolpe et al, 1982a). However, later studies have demonstrated that MPA, in doses adequate for endometrial protection (10 mg) (Gibbons et al, 1986; Whitehead, 1986), antagonizes the oestrogenic actions on HDL-C. Ottosson et al (1985) observed a significant decrease in HDL-C of 8% (and HDL_2-C of 17%) following the addition of 10 mg MPA to postmenopausal women primed with oestrogens (2 mg oestradiol valerate), and the oestrogen-induced rise in HDL-C has been reduced or absent in other studies using corresponding hormone doses (Hirvonen et al, 1987; Haarbo et al, 1991; Marslew et al, 1991b). Similar modifying actions on HDL-C have been observed following cyclic administration of CPA (1 mg) (Jensen et al, 1987a, 1989; Hirvonen et al, 1990), DD (10 mg) (Fletcher et al, 1987) and lower doses of MPA (5 mg) (Sherwin and Gelfand, 1989), but in general these actions may be moderate compared with 19-nortestosterone derivatives. Oestrogen-induced changes in total cholesterol and LDL-C seem virtually unaffected by the addition of 17-hydroxyprogesterone derivatives. It is prudent to note that doses sufficient for endometrial protection have not been defined for most 17-hydroxyprogesterone derivatives and the doses used in these studies may eventually appear to be suboptimal.

As with 19-nortestosterone-derived progestogens, the antagonizing actions of 17-hydroxyprogesterone regimens become more prominent when administered continuously. Thus, continuous combinations of small doses of MPA (2.5 mg and 5 mg), MGA (2.5 mg and 5 mg) and CPA (1 mg) with conventional doses of oestrogens have been reported to abolish the expected oestrogen-induced rise in HDL-C (Prough et al, 1987; Weinstein, 1987; Sporrong et al, 1989; Haarbo et al, 1991; Marslew et al, 1991b).

Only few studies have examined the effects of oral progesterone on lipid metabolism. Fåhreus et al (1983) reported a significant reduction in HDL-C of 10% following the addition of 300 mg progesterone (for 11 days) to postmenopausal women primed with percutaneous oestrogens (3 mg 17β-oestradiol). A smaller dose of progesterone (200 mg for 12 days) added to either percutaneous (Jensen et al, 1987c) or oral oestrogens (Ottosson et al, 1985), however, did not alter any of the oestrogen-induced changes in serum lipids and lipoproteins, and similar findings have been observed following continuous administration of oestradiol (0.7–1.05 mg) and progesterone (200–300 mg) (Hargrove et al, 1989). Hence, it appears that oral progesterone is relatively inert with respect to lipid and lipoprotein metabolism when administered in small, but clinically relevant doses (Lane et al, 1983).

POSTMENOPAUSAL HORMONE REPLACEMENT THERAPY AND CHD

Postmenopausal hormone replacement therapy renders lipid and lipoprotein profiles favourable, but the crucial point is whether these pharmacological changes in lipids and lipoproteins actually reduce the risk of CHD in postmenopausal women.

Several case control and cohort studies have been performed in an attempt to answer this question, but no prospective randomized trial has been performed. Although controversial (Jick et al, 1978; Wilson et al, 1985), the majority of case control and cohort studies (Bain et al, 1981; Ross et al, 1981; Stampfer et al, 1985), including several recent studies (Bush et al, 1987; Henderson et al, 1988; Sullivan et al, 1988), report a reduced risk of CHD in women using postmenopausal oestrogens. The magnitude of protection against CHD varies among the studies, but relative risk odds around or less than 0.5 have been suggested in several studies. In one of the most authoritative studies, The Lipid Research Clinics Program Study (Bush et al, 1987), a cohort of 2270 women aged 40–69 years were followed up for 8.5 years. The age-adjusted relative risk of cardiovascular disease deaths in oestrogen users was 0.34 (95% confidence limits: 0.12 to 0.81) compared with non-users, and about half the reduction in CHD could be explained by oestrogen-induced changes in HDL-C and LDL-C. Hence, epidemiological evidence supports a cardioprotective role for postmenopausal oestrogen replacement therapy; however, it should be stressed that current evidence is almost exclusively based on the use of unopposed oestrogen treatment and that no equivalent data are yet available for the use of combined oestrogen-progestogen therapy. Nevertheless, the data emphasize the importance of judicial selection of an appropriate progestogen for postmenopausal hormone replacement in order to preserve the oestrogenic actions on lipid and lipoprotein metabolism.

SUMMARY

Cardiovascular disease is the leading cause of death in women but manifests itself primarily in the postmenopausal years. Menopause appears to increase the cardiovascular risk, at least when surgically induced, whereas the effects of the natural menopause are still a matter of debate. Why postmenopausal women apparently lose their natural cardioprotection is not established, but oestrogen deficiency seems to play an important role.

Loss of ovarian hormone production at the menopause significantly alters serum lipids and lipoproteins, giving rise to more atherogenic lipid profiles throughout the postmenopausal years, and these changes may in part be responsible for the alleged cardiovascular risk.

Postmenopausal hormone replacement therapy, using oral unopposed oestrogens, induces potential favourable effects on lipids and lipoproteins, and epidemiological evidence has established that the risk of cardiovascular mortality is reduced by 40–60% in women receiving postmenopausal oes-trogen therapy. Part of this reduction seems to be explained by changes in lipids and lipoproteins. Parenteral administration of oestrogens induces comparable, although less pronounced effects on lipids and lipoproteins, and the possible cardioprotective role of parenteral administration remains obscure.

The addition of progestogens to postmenopausal oestrogen therapy is essential for endometrial protection, but progestogens apparently anta-gonize some of the actions of oestrogens on lipid metabolism. However, the type, the dose, the duration and the route of administration, as well as the potency balance between the oestrogen and the progestogen employed, are important determinants for the ultimate effect on lipid metabolism. With the use of cyclic administration and the lowest possible doses of proges-togens, the oestrogenic actions on lipids and lipoproteins can be largely preserved, but the cardioprotective potential of combined oestrogen-progestogen therapy is as yet unknown.

REFERENCES

Adami A, Bertoldo F, Zamberlan N, Gatti D & Carriero PL (1990) Long-term effects of transdermal and oral oestrogen on serum lipoproteins in postmenopausal women. *Abstracts of The Sixth International Congress on the Menopause*, Bangkok, p 238.

Bain C, Willett W, Hennekens CJ et al (1981) Use of postmenopausal hormones and risk of myocardial infarction. *Circulation* **64:** 42–46.

Basdevant A, De Lignieres B & Guy-Grand B (1983) Differential lipemic and hormonal responses to oral and parenteral 17β-oestradiol in postmenopausal women. *American Journal of Obstetrics and Gynecology* **147:** 77–81.

Bengtsson C & Lindquist O (1978) Coronary heart disease during the menopause. In Oliver MF (ed.) *Coronary Heart Disease in Young Women*, pp 234–239. Edinburgh: Churchill Livingstone.

Blanc J-J, Boschat J, Morin J-F, Clavier J & Penther P (1977) Menopause and myocardial infarction. *American Journal of Obstetrics and Gynecology* **127:** 353–355.

Bonithon-Kopp C, Scarabin P-Y, Darne B, Malmejac A & Guize L (1990) Menopause-related changes in lipoproteins and some other cardiovascular risk factors. *International Journal of Epidemiology* **19:** 42–48.

Bush TL, Barrett-Connor S, Cowen LD et al (1987) Cardiovascular mortality and non-contraceptive use of oestrogen in women: results from the Lipid Research Clinics Program Follow-up Study. *Circulation* **75:** 1102–1109.

Bush TL & Miller VT (1987) Effects of pharmacologic agents used during menopause: Impact on lipids and lipoproteins. In Mishell DR Jr (ed.) *Menopause, Physiology and Pharmacology*, pp 187–208. Chicago: Year Book Medical.

Bush T, Cowan L, Heiss G, Chambliss L & Wallace R (1984) Ovarian function and lipid/lipoprotein levels. Results from the Lipid Research Clinics Program. *American Journal of Epidemiology* **120:** 489.

Bush TL, Fried LP & Barrett-Connor E (1988) Cholesterol, lipoproteins, and coronary heart disease in women. *Clinical Chemistry* **34:** B60–B70.

Castelli WP, Garrison RJ, Wilson PWF et al (1986) Incidence of coronary heart disease and lipoprotein cholesterol levels. The Framingham Study. *Journal of the American Medical Association* **256:** 2835–2838.

Chetkowski RJ, Meldrum DR, Steingole KA et al (1986) Biologic effects of transdermal estradiol. *New England Journal of Medicine* **314:** 1615–1620.

Connor SL, Connor WE, Sexton G, Calvin L & Bacon S (1982) The effects of age, body weight and family relationships on plasma lipoproteins and lipids in men, women, and children of randomly selected families. *Circulation* **65:** 1290–1298.

Colditz GA, Willett WC, Stampfer MJ et al (1987) Menopause and the risk of coronary heart disease in women. *New England Journal of Medicine* **316:** 1105–1110.

Consensus Report (1988) Progestagen use in postmenopausal women. *Lancet* **ii:** 1243–1244.

Egeland GM, Kuller LH, Matthews KA et al (1990) Hormone replacement therapy and lipoprotein changes during early menopause. *Obstetrics and Gynecology* **76:** 776–782.

Elkik F, Gompel A, Mercier-Bodard C et al (1982) Effects of percutaneous estradiol and conjugated estrogens on the level of plasma proteins and triglycerides in postmenopausal women. *American Journal of Obstetrics and Gynecology* **143:** 888–892.

Fåhreaus L & Wallentin L (1983) High density lipoprotein subfractions during oral and cutaneous administration of 17β-oestradiol to menopausal women. *Journal of Clinical Endocrinology and Metabolism* **56:** 797–801.

Fåhreaus L, Larsson-Cohn U & Wallentin L (1982) Lipoproteins during oral and cutaneous administration of oestradiol-17β to menopausal women. *Acta Endocrinologica* **101:** 597–602.

Fåhreaus L, Larsson-Cohn U & Wallentin L (1983) L-Norgestrel and progesterone have different influences on plasma lipoproteins. *European Journal of Clinical Investigation* **13:** 447–453.

Farish E, Fletcher CD, Hart DM et al (1984) The effects of hormone implants on serum lipoproteins and steroid hormones in bilaterally oophorectomised women. *Acta Endocrinologica* **106:** 116–120.

Farish E, Fletcher CD, Hart DM et al (1986) The effects of conjugated equine oestrogens with and without a cyclical progestogen on lipoproteins and HDL subfractions in postmenopausal women. *Acta Endocrinologica* **113**: 123–127.

Farish E, Fletcher CH, Dagen MM et al (1989) Lipoprotein and apolipoprotein levels in postmenopausal women on continuous oestrogen/progestogen therapy. *British Journal of Obstetrics and Gynaecology* **96**: 358–364.

Farish E, Fletcher CD, Hart DM & Smith MI (1990) Effects of bilateral oophorectomy on lipoprotein metabolism. *British Journal of Obstetrics and Gynaecology* **97**: 78–82.

Fletcher CD, Farish E, Hart DM et al (1986) Long-term hormone implant therapy—effects on lipoproteins and steroid level in post-menopausal women. *Acta Endocrinologica* **111**: 419–423.

Fletcher CD, Farish E, Dagen MM & Hart DM (1987) A comparison of the effects of lipoproteins of two progestogens used during cyclical hormone replacement therapy. *Maturitas* **9**: 253–258.

Gambrell RD, Bagnell CA & Greenblatt RB (1983) Role of oestrogens and progesterone in the etiology and prevention of endometrial cancer: Review. *American Journal of Obstetrics and Gynecology* **146**: 696–707.

Gibbons WE, Moyer DL, Lobo RA, Roy S & Mishell DR Jr (1986) Biochemical and histologic effects of sequential estrogen/progestin therapy on the endometrium of postmenopausal women. *American Journal of Obstetrics and Gynecology* **154**: 456–461.

Goebelsmann U, Mashchak A & Mishell DR (1985) Comparison of hepatic impact of oral and vaginal administration of ethinyl estradiol. *American Journal of Obstetrics and Gynecology* **151**: 868–877.

Gordon T, Castelli WP, Hjortland NMC & Kannel WB (1977a) The prediction of coronary heart disease by high-density and other lipoproteins: An historical perspective. In Rifkind BM & Levy RI (eds) *Hyperlipidemia, Diagnosis and Therapy*, pp 71–78. New York: Grune & Stratton.

Gordon T, Castelli WP, Hjortland MC, Kannel WB & Dawber TR (1977b) High density lipoproteins as a protective factor against coronary heart disease. The Framingham Study. *American Journal of Medicine* **62**: 707–714.

Gordon T, Kannel WB, Hjortland MC & McNamara PM (1978) Menopause and coronary heart disease. The Framingham Study. *Annals of Internal Medicine* **89**: 157–161.

Haarbo J, Hassager C, Jensen SB, Riis BJ & Christiansen C (1991) Serum lipids, lipoproteins, and apolipoproteins during postmenopausal estrogen replacement therapy combined with either 19-nortestosterone derivatives or 17-hydroxyprogesterone derivatives. *American Journal of Medicine* **90**: 584–589.

Hammond CB, Jelovsek FR, Lee KL, Creasman WT & Parker RT (1979) Effects of long-term estrogen replacement therapy. II. Neoplasia. *American Journal of Obstetrics and Gynecology* **133**: 537–547.

Hargrove JT, Maxon WS, Wentz AC & Burnett LS (1989) Menopausal hormone replacement therapy with continuous daily oral micronized estradiol and progesterone. *Obstetrics and Gynecology* **73**: 606–612.

Heiss G, Tamir I, Davis CE et al (1980) Lipoprotein-cholesterol distributions in selected North American populations: The Lipid Research Clinics Program Prevalence Study. *Circulation* **61**: 302–315.

Henderson BE, Paganini-Hill A & Ross RK (1988) Estrogen replacement therapy and protection from acute myocardial infarction. *American Journal of Obstetrics and Gynecology* **159**: 312–317.

Hirvonen E, Mälkönen M & Manninen V (1981) Effects of different progestogens on lipoproteins during postmenopausal replacement therapy. *New England Journal of Medicine* **304**: 560–563.

Hirvonen E, Lipasti A, Mälkönen M et al (1987) Clinical and lipid metabolic effects of unopposed oestrogen and two oestrogen-progestogen regimens in postmenopausal women. *Maturitas* **9**: 69–79.

Hirvonen E, Elliesen J & Schmidt-Gollwitzer K (1990) Comparison of two hormone replacement regimens—influence on lipoproteins and bone mineral content. *Maturitas* **12**: 127–136.

Hjortland MC, McNamara PM & Kannel WB (1976) Some atherogenic concomitants of menopause: The Framingham Study. *American Journal of Epidemiology* **103**: 304–311.

Holst J, Cajander S, Carlström K, Damber M-G & von Schoultz B (1983) A comparison of liver protein induction in postmenopausal women during oral and percutaneous oestrogen replacement therapy. *British Journal of Obstetrics and Gynaecology* **90**: 355–360.

Hulley SB, Rosenman RH, Bawol RD & Brand RJ (1980) Epidemiology as a guide to clinical decisions. The association between triglycerides and coronary heart disease. *New England Journal of Medicine* **302**: 1383–1389.

Jensen J, Nilas L & Christiansen C (1986) Cyclic changes in serum cholesterol and lipoproteins following different doses of combined postmenopausal hormone replacement therapy. *British Journal of Obstetrics and Gynaecology* **92**: 613–618.

Jensen J & Christiansen C (1987) Dose-response effects on serum lipids and lipoproteins following combined oestrogen-progestogen therapy in postmenopausal women. *Maturitas* **9**: 259–266.

Jensen J, Riis BJ & Christiansen C (1987a) Cyproterone acetate, an alternative progestogen in postmenopausal hormone replacement therapy? Effects on serum lipids and lipoproteins. *British Journal of Obstetrics and Gynaecology* **94**: 136–141.

Jensen J, Riis BJ, Strøm V & Christiansen C (1987b) Continuous oestrogen-progestogen treatment and serum lipoproteins in postmenopausal women. *British Journal of Obstetrics and Gynaecology* **94**: 130–135.

Jensen J, Riis BJ, Strøm V, Nilas L & Christiansen C (1987c) Long-term effects of percutaneous estrogens and oral progesterone on serum lipoproteins in postmenopausal women. *American Journal of Obstetrics and Gynecology* **156**: 66–71.

Jensen J, Riis BJ, Strøm V & Christiansen C (1989) Long-term and withdrawal effects of two different oestrogen-progestogen combinations on lipid and lipoprotein profiles in postmenopausal women. *Maturitas* **11**: 117–128.

Jensen J, Nilas L & Christiansen C (1990) The influence of menopause on serum lipids and lipoproteins. *Maturitas* **12**: 321–331.

Jick H, Dinan B & Rothman KJ (1978) Noncontraceptive estrogens and nonfatal myocardial infarction. *Journal of the American Medical Association* **239**: 1407–1408.

Kannel WB & Gordon T (1987) Cardiovascular effects of the menopause. In Mishell DR Jr (ed.) *Menopause, Physiology and Pharmacology*, pp 91–102. New York: Year Book Medical.

Kannel WB, Castelli WP, Gordon T & McNamara PM (1971) Serum cholesterol, lipoproteins, and the risk of coronary heart disease. The Framingham Study. *Annals of Internal Medicine* **74**: 1–12.

Kissebah AH, Harrigan P & Wynn V (1973) Mechanism of hypertriglyceridaemia associated with contraceptive steroids. *Hormone and Metabolic Research* **5**: 184–190.

Klorfajn I, Mizrahy O & Assa S (1978) A study on serum lipids of the elderly. *Journal of Gerontology* **33**: 48–51.

Kovanen PT, Brown MS & Goldstein JL (1979) Increased binding of low density lipoprotein to liver membranes from rats treated with 17α-ethinyl estradiol. *Journal of Biological Chemistry* **254**: 11367–11373.

Krauss RM, Perlman JA, Ray R & Petitti D (1988) Effects of estrogen dose and smoking on lipid and lipoprotein levels in postmenopausal women. *American Journal of Obstetrics and Gynecology* **158**: 1606–1611.

Lagrelius A, Fredricsson B, Hirt M & Weintraub L (1986) Clinical experience with a low-dose combination of estradiol valerate and levonorgestrel. *Acta Obstetrica et Gynecologica Scandinavica* **134**: 97–101.

Lane G, Siddle NC, Ryder TA et al (1983) Dose dependent effects of oral progesterone on the oestrogenized postmenopausal endometrium. *British Medical Journal* **287**: 1241–1245.

Lapidus L, Bengtsson C & Lindquist O (1985a) Menopausal age and risk of cardiovascular disease and death. *Acta Obstetrica et Gynecologica Scandinavica* **130**: 37–41.

Lapidus L, Bengtsson C, Lindquist O, Sigurdsson JA & Rybo E (1985b) Triglycerides—main lipid risk factor for cardiovascular disease in women? *Acta Medica Scandinavica* **217**: 481–489.

Lindgren R, Berg G, Hammar M, Larsson-Cohn U & Olsson AG (1990) Plasma lipids and lipoproteins in climacteric women treated with sequential transdermal patches containing 17β-oestradiol and 17β-oestradiol/norethisterone. *Abstracts of The Sixth International Congress on the Menopause*, Bangkok, p 282.

Lindquist O (1982) Intraindividual changes of blood pressure, serum lipids, and body weight in relation to menstrual status: Results from a prospective population study of women in Göteborg. *Preventive Medicine* **11**: 162–172.

Lindquist O & Bengtsson C (1980) Serum lipids, arterial blood pressure and body weight in relation to the menopause: results from a population study of women in Göteborg, Sweden. *Scandinavian Journal of Clinical and Laboratory Investigation* **40**: 629–636.

Lipid Research Clinics Program (1984) The Lipid Research Clinics Coronary Primany Prevention Trial Results. II. The relationship of reduction in incidence of coronary heart disease to cholesterol lowering. *Journal of the American Medical Association* **251**: 365–374.

Manchester JH, Herman MV & Gorlin RG (1971) Premenopausal castration and documented coronary atherosclerosis. *American Journal of Cardiology* **28**: 33–37.

Mandel FP, Geola FL, Meldrum DR et al (1983) Biological effects of various doses of vaginally administered conjugated equine estrogens in postmenopausal women. *Journal of Clinical Endocrinology and Metabolism* **57**: 133–139.

Marslew U, Riis BJ & Christiansen C (1991a) Desogestrel in hormone replacement therapy: Long-term effects on bone, calcium and lipid metabolism, climacteric symptoms, and bleeding. *European Journal of Clinical Investigation* (in press).

Marslew U, Overgaard K, Riis BJ & Christiansen C (1991b) Two new combinations of oestrogen and progestogen for prevention of postmenopausal bone loss. Long-term effects on bone, calcium and lipid metabolism, climacteric symptoms, and bleeding. *British Journal of Obstetrics and Gynaecology* (in press).

Martin MJ, Hulley SB, Browner WS, Kuller LH & Wenthworth D (1986) Serum cholesterol, blood pressure, and mortality: Implications from a cohort of 361 662 men. *Lancet* **ii**: 933–936.

Matthews KA, Milahn E, Kuller LH et al (1989) Menopause and risk factors for coronary heart disease. *New England Journal of Medicine* **321**: 641–646.

Mattsson L-Å, Cullberg G & Samsioe G (1982) Evaluation of a continuous oestrogen-progestogen regimen for climacteric complaints. *Maturitas* **4**: 95–102.

Mattsson L, Cullberg G & Samsioe G (1984) A continuous estrogen-progestogen regimen for climacteric complaints. Effects on lipid and lipoprotein metabolism. *Acta Obstetrica et Gynecologica Scandinavica* **63**: 673–677.

Miller NE (1987) Associations of high-density lipoprotein subclasses and apolipoproteins with ischaemic heart disease and coronary atherosclerosis. *American Heart Journal* **113**: 589–597.

Miller NE, Førde OH, Thelle DS & Mjøs OD (1977) The Tromsø Heart Study. High density lipoprotein and coronary heart disease: A prospective case-control study. *Lancet* **i**: 965–968.

Notelovitz M, Gudat JC, Ware MD & Dougherty MC (1982) Oestrogen-progestin therapy and the lipid balance of post-menopausal women. *Maturitas* **4**: 301–308.

Ottosson UB, Johansson BG & von Schoultz B (1985) Subfractions of high-density lipoprotein cholesterol during estrogen replacement therapy: A comparison between progestogens and natural progesterone. *American Journal of Obstetrics and Gynecology* **151**: 746–750.

Persson IR, Adami H-O, Eklund G et al (1986) The risk of endometrial neoplasia and treatment with estrogen-progestogen combinations. *Acta Obstetrica et Gynecologica Scandinavica* **65**: 211–217.

Prough SG, Aksel S, Wiebe RH & Shepherd J (1987) Continuous estrogen/progestin therapy in menopause. *American Journal of Obstetrics and Gynecology* **157**: 1449–1453.

Rijpkema AHM, van der Sanden AA & Ruijs AHC (1990) Effects of post-menopausal oestrogen-progestogen replacement therapy on serum lipids and lipoproteins: a review. *Maturitas* **12**: 259–285.

Rosenberg L, Hennekens CH, Rosner B et al (1981) Early menopause and the risk of myocardial infarction. *American Journal of Obstetrics and Gynecology* **139**: 47–51.

Ross FK, Paganini-Hill A, Mack TM, Arthur M & Henderson BE (1981) Menopausal oestrogen therapy and protection from death from ischaemic heart disease. *Lancet* **i**: 858–860.

Schaefer EJ, Foster DM, Zech LA et al (1983) The effects of estrogen administration on plasma lipoprotein metabolism in premenopausal females. *Journal of Clinical Endocrinology and Metabolism* **57**: 262–267.

Sharf M, Oettinger M, Lanir A, Kahana L & Yeshurun D (1985) Lipid and lipoprotein levels following pure estradiol implantation in post-menopausal women. *Gynecologic and Obstetric Investigation* **19**: 207–212.

Sherwin BB & Gelfand MM (1989) A prospective one-year study of estrogen and progestin in postmenopausal women: Effects on clinical symptoms and lipoprotein lipids. *Obstetrics and Gynecology* **73**: 759–766.

Sherwin BB, Gelfand MM, Schucher R & Gabor J (1987) Postmenopausal estrogen and androgen replacement and lipoprotein lipid concentrations. *American Journal of Obstetrics and Gynecology* **156**: 414–419.

Siddle NC, Townsend PT, Young O et al (1982) Dose-dependent effects of synthetic progestins on the biochemistry of the estrogenized post-menopausal endometrium. *Acta Obstetrica et Gynecologica Scandinavica* **106(supplement)**: 17–22.

Silverstolpe G, Gustafson A, Samsioe G & Svanborg A (1982a) Lipid metabolic studies in oophorectomised women: effects on serum lipids and lipoproteins of three synthetic progestogens. *Maturitas* **4**: 103–111.

Silverstolpe G, Gustafson A, Samsioe G & Svanborg A (1982b) Lipid and carbohydrate metabolism studies in oophorectomized women: Effects produced by the addition of norethisterone acetate to two estrogen preparations. *Archives of Gynecology* **231**: 279–287.

Sporrong T, Hellgren M, Samsioe G & Mattsson L-Å (1989) Metabolic effects of continuous estradiol-progestin therapy in postmenopausal women. *Obstetrics and Gynecology* **73**: 754–758.

Staland B (1981) Continuous treatment with natural oestrogens and progestogens. A way of avoiding endometrial stimulation. *Maturitas* **3**: 145–156.

Stampfer MJ, Willett WC, Colditz GA et al (1985) A prospective study of postmenopausal estrogen therapy and coronary heart disease. *New England Journal of Medicine* **313**: 1044–1049.

Stanczyk FZ, Shoupe D, Nunez V et al (1988) A randomized comparison of nonoral estradiol delivery in postmenopausal women. *American Journal of Obstetrics and Gynecology* **159**: 1540–1546.

Sullivan JM, Zwaag RV, Lemp GF et al (1988) Postmenopausal estrogen use and coronary atherosclerosis. *Annals of Internal Medicine* **108**: 358–363.

Tikkanen MJ, Kuusi T, Nikkilä EA & Sipinen S (1986) Post-menopausal hormone replacement therapy: effects of progestogens on serum lipids and lipoproteins. A review. *Maturitas* **8**: 7–17.

Tyroler HA (1987) Review of lipid-lowering clinical trial in relation to observational epidemiologic studies. *Circulation* **76**: 515–522.

Weinstein L (1987) Efficacy of a continuous estrogen-progestin regimen in the menopausal patient. *Obstetrics and Gynecology* **69**: 929–932.

Whitehead MI (1986) Prevention of endometrial abnormalities. *Acta Obstetrica et Gynecologica Scandinavica* **134(supplement)**: 81–91.

Whitehead MI, Townsend PT, Pryse-Davies J, Ryder TA & King RJB (1981) Effects of estrogens and progestins on the biochemistry and morphology of the postmenopausal endometrium. *New England Journal of Medicine* **305**: 1599–1605.

Wilson PWF, Garrison RJ & Castelli WP (1985) Postmenopausal estrogen use, cigarette smoking, and cardiovascular morbidity in women over 50. The Framingham Study. *New England Journal of Medicine* **313**: 1038–1043.

Witteman JCM, Grobbee DE, Kok FJ, Hofman A & Valkenburg HA (1989) Increased risk of atherosclerosis in women after the menopause. *British Medical Journal* **298**: 642–644.

9

Oestrogen therapy and cardiovascular disease: do the benefits outweigh the risks?

TRUDY L. BUSH
KATHERINE MILLER-BASS

In all developed countries, cardiovascular disease (CVD) is the leading cause of death in women past the age of menopause, accounting for nearly twice as many deaths as all cancers combined. The numbers of women who succumb prematurely to CVD are quite high. In the United States, for example 130 000 women aged 50–74 years die from CVD each year compared with 23 000 who die from breast cancer, 29 000 who die from lung cancer, or 750 who die from osteoporosis-related hip fractures (National Center for Health Statistics, 1990). CVD is also a leading cause of morbidity and disability in women (Fried et al, 1987), and accounts for tremendous expenditure in health costs (Havlik et al, 1987).

Oestrogen replacement therapy in peri- and postmenopausal women has traditionally been used for the relief of postmenopausal symptoms (such as hot flushes and urogenital atrophy) and for the prevention of osteoporosis (Notelovitz, 1989). These benefits of oestrogen therapy are well known, as is the one documented risk (endometrial cancer) (Henderson, 1989). However, the beneficial cardiovascular effects of oestrogen therapy are less well recognized, despite the relatively large and growing body of literature showing that oestrogen use significantly reduces a woman's risk of CVD (Bush, 1990). In fact, a substantial number of physicians and other health care providers believe that oestrogen use increases a woman's risk of CVD.

One reason that the positive cardiovascular effects of oestrogen replacement therapy are not well known is because menopausal oestrogen therapy is still confused with oral contraceptive therapy. While oral contraceptive use is still considered to increase a woman's risk of a cardiovascular event (particularly if she smokes), a clear distinction must be made between contraceptive and non-contraceptive therapy. Oral contraceptives contain relatively high doses of a synthetic oestrogen and a 19-nor-progestin, while non-contraceptive therapy is usually low dose, natural oestrogen with or without a low androgenic progestin.

If postmenopausal oestrogen therapy is indeed cardioprotective, then, given the importance of CVD for women, this benefit would far outweigh any known (i.e. endometrial cancer) or perceived (i.e. breast cancer) risks of use. Given this background, the purpose of this chapter is threefold: one,

Baillière's Clinical Obstetrics and Gynaecology—
Vol. 5, No. 4, December 1991
ISBN 0–7020–1548–2

to review briefly the indications, complications and current modes of administration of oestrogen replacement therapy; two, to review the epidemiological evidence on the association between oestrogen therapy and CVD in women; and three, to examine the relevance of the route of oestrogen administration and the effects of concurrent progestin administration with oestrogen therapy on cardioprotection. These last two topics are areas of considerable controversy at this time.

OESTROGEN REPLACEMENT THERAPY

Overview

In the United States, oestrogen replacement therapy (including oestrogen/ progestin combinations) is currently approved only for the amelioration of menopausal symptoms and for the prevention of osteoporosis. Progestins are prescribed with oestrogens, either continuously or cyclically, to prevent oestrogen-induced endometrial hyperplasia and carcinoma in women with an intact uterus. Oestrogen and oestrogen/progestin use is relatively common in the United States; a recent survey in an upper middle class community in California found that up to one-third of women aged 50 to 65 years were currently taking oestrogen or oestrogen-progestin therapy (Harris et al, 1990). This is in contrast to the patterns seen in Europe, where oestrogen (and oestrogen/progestin) use is reported less frequently (5–15%) (Thompson et al, 1989; Van Der Giezen et al, 1990).

Both oral and parenteral forms of oestrogen are available, although in practice, oral therapy is far and away the most widely used in the United States (Miller-Bass and Adashi, 1990). The vast majority of oral oestrogens prescribed are conjugated equine oestrogens (Premarin, made by Wyeth-Ayerst Laboratories, Philadelphia, Pennsylvania) (Miller-Bass and Adashi, 1990); because of this, nearly all studies which have examined the effect of oestrogen on CVD risk have evaluated conjugated equine oestrogens.

Other oral oestrogens used in the United States and in other countries include diethylstilbesterol (DES), micronized 17β-oestradiol (Estrace, made by Mead Johnson Laboratories, Evansville, Indiana), piperazine oestrone sulphate (estropipate USP) (Ogen, made by Abbott Pharmaceuticals, North Chicago, Illinois), and 17α-ethinyloestradiol (Estinyl, made by Schering Corporation, Kenilworth, New Jersey). Unfortunately, few data on the direct cardiovascular effects of these oral agents are currently available.

Parenteral forms of oestrogen include vaginal creams, percutaneous gels, injectable oestrogens, subcutaneous pellets, and intranasal and sublingual preparations. Vaginal oestrogen creams are used primarily for the relief of local symptoms related to postmenopausal vaginal atrophy. Percutaneous oestradiol gel is used commonly in Europe; however, it is not commercially available in the United States at this time. Injectable oestrogens, while available and occasionally used, are quickly absorbed and metabolized after administration, making them impractical for long-term therapy (Stumpf,

1990). Subcutaneous oestradiol pellets have been extensively studied, but are not commercially marketed in the United States. Additionally, they have the disadvantage of requiring minor surgical procedures for insertion and removal. Intranasal and sublingual oestrogen preparations are currently used only for research purposes (Miller-Bass and Adashi, 1990).

The major non-oral oestrogen used in the United States is a transdermal oestradiol, available in the form of a transdermal therapeutic system, or patch, and marketed under the trade name of Estraderm (made by Ciba-Geigy Pharmaceuticals, Summit, New Jersey). The patch has been available for a few years and may be gaining acceptance among patients and practitioners. Unfortunately, this mode of therapy has not been used frequently enough or long enough for studies of the direct effects on CVD to be completed.

Indications

As noted previously, the indications for oestrogen therapy fall into three general categories: relief of vasomotor, genitourinary and psychological symptoms; prevention of osteoporosis; and cardioprotection (Notelovitz, 1989). Cardioprotection is discussed in detail in the latter portion of this chapter, and osteoporosis is discussed elsewhere in this issue. Thus, the use of oestrogens for relief of menopausal symptoms is addressed briefly here.

Menopausal symptoms

By far the most common symptom for which menopausal women seek treatment is the hot flush (Judd et al, 1983). It is estimated that these episodes of flushing and perspiration will occur in more than 80% of menopausal women, and will persist for at least 1 year in a similar percentage (Judd et al, 1983; Notelovitz, 1989). Hot flushes can be effectively treated with oral or parenteral oestrogen therapy. Oral administration of standard doses of both conjugated equine oestrogens (0.625 mg/day) and micronized 17β-oestradiol (2 mg/day) has been demonstrated to significantly decrease subjectively recorded hot flushes in menopausal women (Martin et al, 1972; Callantine et al, 1975; Coope et al, 1975). Similarly, hot flushes are relieved by oestradiol delivered transdermally, percutaneously or by subcutaneous pellet (Holst et al, 1983; Padwick et al, 1985; Stanczyk et al, 1988).

Urogenital atrophy occurs in virtually all postmenopausal women and because such atrophic changes can result in dyspareunia, vaginal infections and dysuria (Notelovitz, 1989), many women seek medical attention for this problem. Both oral and parenteral administration of oestrogen can reverse the atrophic changes and provide relief of symptoms. Vaginal oestrogen creams containing as little as 0.3 mg/dl of conjugated oestrogens can successfully reverse atrophic vaginal changes (Mandel et al, 1983). At standard doses, orally administered conjugated equine oestrogens, micronized 17β-oestradiol and ethinyloestradiol can revert the vaginal epithelium to a premenopausal state (Martin et al, 1972; Geola et al, 1980; Mandel et al,

1982), as can transdermal oestradiol (Laufer et al, 1983; Padwick et al, 1985; Chetkowski et al, 1986; Haas et al, 1988), relieving some of the symptoms of atrophy.

Many psychological changes, including insomnia, irritability and depression, are reportedly associated with the menopause (Notelovitz, 1989), and while some of these, such as insomnia, are clearly related to concurrent vasomotor symptoms and will improve when hot flushes are abolished (Ravnikar, 1990), others are less easily explained. However, many patients report significant improvement in these psychological symptoms, as well as an increased feeling of 'well-being', during treatment with either oral or parenteral oestrogen preparations (Martin et al, 1972; Coope et al, 1975; Campbell and Whitehead, 1977; Padwick et al, 1985).

Complications

Despite the non-cardiovascular benefits of oestrogen therapy outlined above, considerable concern exists regarding the risks of oestrogen therapy. This concern is expressed by the observation that a large proportion of women for whom oestrogen may be indicated are not prescribed or refuse to take this therapy (Hemminki et al, 1988). The risks or complications of oestrogen therapy can be divided into two main groups: those related to the hepatic, or 'first-pass', metabolism of oral oestrogen therapy, and those related to neoplasia, particularly endometrial and breast cancer.

Hepatic effects

One of the major disadvantages of oral oestrogen therapy is the marked 'first-pass' hepatic metabolism that occurs when these oestrogens are delivered directly to the liver via the portal circulation following their absorption from the intestines. The result is enhanced protein synthesis and altered lipid metabolism in the liver, and many of the undesirable (and perhaps undocumented) side-effects of oestrogen therapy, such as hypertension, hypercoagulability and cholelithiasis, are thought to be secondary to this first-pass phenomenon (Cedars and Judd, 1987; Miller-Bass and Adashi, 1990).

Oral administration of standard doses of conjugated equine oestrogens, micronized 17β-oestradiol, ethinyloestradiol and oestrone sulphate have been shown to lead to significant increases in the hepatic proteins, including corticosteroid-binding globulin, thyroid-binding globulin, sex hormone-binding globulin and renin substrate (Geola et al, 1980; Mandel et al, 1982; Mashchak et al, 1982). Even vaginal conjugated equine oestrogen preparations, at high enough doses, will lead to increases in hepatic protein synthesis (Mandel et al, 1982; Goebelsmann et al, 1985), probably by absorption into the systemic bloodstream. Oestrogen therapy also alters hepatic lipid metabolism, and changes in bile acids noted in women on oestrogen therapy have been proposed as the mechanism responsible for the increased incidence of gallbladder disease seen in these women (Boston Collaborative Drug Surveillance Program, 1974; Cedars and Judd, 1987).

While there continues to be some concern that oestrogen therapy may be responsible for the development or exacerbation of hypertension in women, the overall effect of oestrogen on blood pressure appears to be a slight lowering of both the systolic and diastolic pressures (Luotola, 1983; Lobo, 1989, 1990; Barrett-Connor, 1990). However, there appear to be susceptible individuals in whom oestrogen administration may lead to increases in blood pressure (Lobo, 1989; Barrett-Connor, 1990). The mechanism for this is thought to be related to changes in the renin-angiotensin system, specifically increases in renin substrate, which have been noted following oral oestrogen therapy (Cedars and Judd, 1987).

The effects of orally administered oestrogens on the liver may also result in altered levels of those clotting factors which are hepatic in origin, such as factors VII, IX and X (Cedars and Judd, 1987). However, controlled experiments and observational studies have not demonstrated any increase in thrombophlebitis associated with menopausal oestrogen therapy (Boston Collaborative Drug Surveillance Program, 1974).

A major benefit of non-oral routes of oestrogen therapy is their limited first-pass metabolism, a feature which should lead to a reduction in the incidence of some of the complications of oestrogen therapy noted above. While vaginal administration of conjugated equine oestrogens and ethinyloestradiol at relatively high doses has been noted to result in significantly enhanced liver protein synthesis (Mandel et al, 1983; Goebelsmann et al, 1985), this has not been the case at the lower doses which can effectively reverse atrophic vaginal changes, nor have similar changes been demonstrated with other parenteral forms of oestrogen therapy. The administration of standard doses of either transdermal (Laufer et al, 1983; Padwick et al, 1985; Chetkowski et al, 1986; Haas et al, 1988) or percutaneous (Holst et al, 1983; De Lignieres et al, 1986) 17β-oestradiol has been shown to result in only minimal and non-significant increases in hepatic proteins. Similarly, no increase in hepatic protein synthesis was observed during the use of subcutaneous oestradiol pellets (25 mg) (Lobo et al, 1980). Transdermal (Chetkowski et al, 1986) and percutaneous (De Lignieres et al, 1986) preparations have also been demonstrated to lead to no appreciable alterations in the levels of a number of clotting factors, including high molecular weight fibrinogen, fibrinopeptide A and antithrombin III. Antithrombin III activity also remains unchanged.

Unfortunately, there is little published information regarding the actual effects of parenteral oestrogen therapy on blood pressure or thrombophlebitis (Barrett-Connor, 1990); however, several investigators have reported either no change (Selby and Peacock, 1986; Haas et al, 1988) or small but non-significant decreases (Padwick et al, 1985) in blood pressure in patients using transdermal oestradiol.

Cancer

The hypothesis that hormones cause cancer is not new, and may be traced to early observations that reproductive factors were associated with differential cancer risk (Lipsett, 1986). For example, it was known as early as the

17th century that nuns, compared with married women, have a higher risk of breast cancer. Thus it has been postulated that pregnancy confers protection against breast cancer.

Although reproductive factors (e.g. nulliparity, age at first pregnancy, age at menarche) have been shown to be related to cancer occurrence, particularly breast and endometrial cancers, the specific endogenous hormonal environments which influence these risks have yet to be determined. In fact, there is continued controversy as to why early pregnancy protects against breast cancer. While oestrogens and progestins are thought to be the major hormones associated with differential cancer risk, other hormones, including dehydroepiandrosterone (DHEA) and prolactin, may also be involved (Gordon et al, 1990).

While reproductive factors, which may include endogenous oestrogens and progestins, are related to the development of reproductive cancers in women, it is inappropriate to assume that exogenous oestrogens and progestins commonly used by women for menopausal treatment are necessarily associated with cancer occurrence. To address the question of whether exogenous oestrogens and progestins cause or prevent cancer, direct studies of women are needed.

Some researchers suggest that hormones, specifically oestrogens, cause or induce cancer by increasing the mitotic rate in target organs, particularly breast tissue, but also germ cells (Henderson et al, 1988b). In fact, exogenous oestrogens do induce mammary cancer in mice, although this effect has not been reported in other species. Furthermore, it has been proposed that progestins may protect against cancer because of their anti-oestrogenic effects: (a) they increase the intracellular conversion of oestradiol (a potent oestrogen) to oestrone (a less active oestrogen), and (b) they slow the rate of translocation of receptor-bound oestradiol to the nucleus, thereby blocking oestrogen's mitotic effects (Henderson et al, 1988b).

The general consensus of the scientific community at this time is that natural oestrogens, if they are associated with an increased cancer occurrence, would act as tumour promoters rather than initiators or true carcinogens (Porter et al, 1987). The major exception is DES, which has been shown to be a tumour initiator. However, DES is a non-steroidal synthetic oestrogen, and may behave differently compared to natural steroidal oestrogens. At this time, relatively little is known about the potential of progestins in the absence of oestrogens to induce, promote or suppress carcinogenesis.

Currently, there is well-accepted evidence that exogenous oestrogen use is associated with an increase in two specific tumours: vaginal cancer in the daughters of women who used DES during pregnancy, and endometrial tumours in women who used unopposed oestrogen therapy for menopausal symptoms. The data on oestrogens and progestins and endometrial cancers is reviewed here briefly; the evidence that breast tumours are increased or decreased by oestrogen and/or progestin use is more controversial and is also evaluated below.

Endometrial cancer. Unopposed oestrogen use is associated with an increased risk of endometrial cancer that is somewhere between two and 12 times that of non-users (Henderson et al, 1989). Since the early case reports of endometrial cancer in oestrogen users in the 1960s, case control and cohort studies have documented this association (Judd et al, 1983; Henderson, 1988b). Some researchers have questioned the validity of the reports from the case control studies, but the current scientific consensus is that the data reflect a true and causal association. One explanation for the wide variation in the magnitude of risk estimates is that there are frequently large differences in study design and definition of exposure.

The risk of oestrogen-induced endometrial cancer is significantly elevated after 2 to 4 years of treatment and continues to increase to approximately a 10-fold increase after 10 years of use. The risk returns to baseline within 2 years after stopping the treatment (Whitehead and Fraser, 1987). Most studies suggest that the risk is related to both the dose of oestrogen and the duration of use (Henderson, 1989; Notelovitz, 1989; Whitehead et al, 1990).

Conjugated equine oestrogens at doses greater than 1 mg/day are associated with a two-fold higher risk compared with lower doses. However, endometrial cancers which develop in oestrogen users are usually of low stage and grade (Hulka et al, 1980; Judd et al, 1983; Henderson, 1989). In fact, several investigators have reported better survival rates in oestrogen users who develop endometrial cancer than in non-users who develop endometrial cancer (Collins et al, 1980; Henderson, 1989). It has been proposed that the constellation of findings of a short latency period, rapid decline in risk after cessation of use, and biologically less aggressive tumours suggests that oestrogen acts on this tumour by promotion rather than initiation (Henderson et al, 1988b).

The addition of a progestin to oestrogen therapy has been clearly demonstrated to reduce both the incidence of endometrial hyperplasia and the risk of endometrial cancer in oestrogen users (Mishell, 1989; Persson et al, 1989; Whitehead et al, 1990). Duration of progestin treatment may be more important than the actual dose of progestin: in one study, increasing the duration of progestin use from 7 days to 12 days each month reduced the incidence of endometrial hyperplasia from approximately 4% to zero (Whitehead et al, 1990). Unfortunately, many patients on sequential oestrogen–progestin therapy experience monthly bleeding (Notelovitz, 1989; Whitehead et al, 1990), making this therapy unacceptable to some. Other frequently reported side-effects of progestin therapy include bloating, breast tenderness, irritability and depression (Whitehead et al, 1990), as well as possible adverse effects on serum lipids (discussed later). The optimal form and duration of progestin treatment has yet to be conclusively established. However, the Postmenopausal Estrogen/Progestin Interventions (PEPI) trial which is underway in the United States may provide more definitive answers in a few years.

Breast cancer. The effect of oestrogen therapy on the risk of breast cancer is currently an area of some controversy (Whitehead and Fraser, 1987). It seems inherently logical that oestrogen would be associated with an increased risk of breast cancer, since breast tissue is oestrogen sensitive, and since many factors related to endogenous oestrogens (i.e. oophorectomy, late age at menarche, late age at first birth) are also risk factors for breast cancer. However, many studies, even large ones, have found no evidence for an association.

Based on their readings of the data, some researchers have now concluded that oestrogens, particularly long-term oestrogen therapy, leads to a moderate increase in the risk of breast cancer (Henderson, 1989). In a recent review, Henderson (1989) estimates that oestrogen users are subject to an approximately 75% increase in their risk of breast cancer following more than 15 years of use, and that certain subgroups of women (e.g. those with a positive family history) are more susceptible than others. Two recently published and well-publicized studies also appear to support the association of an increased risk of breast cancer in oestrogen users (Bergkvist et al, 1989a; Colditz et al, 1990).

However, these studies and others assessing this association have been subject to considerable criticism due to methodological problems (Whitehead and Fraser, 1987; Henderson, 1989). One major methodological issue is the fact that women taking oestrogens are under the care of physicians, and thus would be more likely to have a tumour diagnosed than women not in the health care system (surveillance bias). Of particular concern in these two well-publicized articles are: (a) the small number of cases and lack of statistical significance in the Swedish study (Bergkvist et al, 1989a), and (b) the strong possibility of surveillance bias in the Nurses' Health Study (Colditz et al, 1990).

While some researchers are convinced that oestrogens increase the risk of breast cancer, others have provided evidence that any increase is quite small. A recent formal meta-analysis of the published data on oestrogen therapy and breast cancer shows only a very slight increase overall (relative risk $= 1.1$) in breast cancer incidence among oestrogen users (DuPont and Page, 1991). Further, this analysis showed no increased risk of breast cancer when the dose of oestrogen was taken into account, and a variable effect of duration of use.

Many patients and physicians are somewhat comforted by the fact that no clear exogenous oestrogen–breast cancer association has yet been documented, despite the fact that menopausal oestrogens have been used for nearly 50 years (Bush and Barrett-Connor, 1985). In comparison, a clear exogenous oestrogen-endometrial cancer association was evident in the 1970s. This failure to find a clear and compelling association suggests that any increase in breast cancer risk in oestrogen users must be small.

In parallel with the evidence seen with endometrial cancer, there is some preliminary indication that oestrogen users who develop breast cancer may have a significantly improved survival compared with non-users who develop breast cancer (Bergkvist et al, 1989b). In fact, several studies have now reported a reduction in mortality from breast cancer among oestrogen users (Gambrell, 1990). These specific findings may reflect surveillance bias, since oestrogen users, who are under the care of physicians, may be more likely to have their tumours diagnosed earlier (at a stage where they are more curable).

An alternative biological hypothesis is that oestrogen promotes the growth of in situ tumours so that they are diagnosed earlier (prior to metastasis). This latter hypothesis might explain the apparent paradoxical findings of an increase in breast cancer incidence but a lowered mortality in users.

Some investigators have interpreted the protective effects of sequential progestogen therapy on the risk of endometrial cancer in oestrogen therapy users to suggest that progestins should be similarly protective for breast cancer. However, there is evidence that the reverse may be true (Bergkvist et al, 1989a). The Swedish study of Bergkvist et al (1989a) demonstrated a (non-significant) higher incidence of breast cancer in women using oestrogen and progestin than in women using oestrogen alone. Concurrently, these authors also reported that women who used oestrogen and progestin and developed breast cancer had a longer survival than women not using oestrogens or using only unopposed oestrogens (Bergkvist et al, 1989b). Despite the results of this one small study, the overall lack of evidence on oestrogen–progestin effects on breast cancer risk means that the actual role of progestogens in breast cancer occurrence remains to be defined.

OESTROGEN REPLACEMENT THERAPY AND CVD

As noted previously, there is a growing body of evidence that oestrogen therapy as described above may also protect against the development of CVD in women. Since there are a large number of published studies examining the association between oestrogen use and CVD, it is useful to have a framework from which to critically examine this literature. One approach is to group the published studies by study design, because design influences both the inferences that can be drawn from a particular study (Bush, 1990) and the 'weight' the study can be given in either a qualitative or quantitative analysis (see Table 1).

In general, experimental studies or clinical trials are considered to be the most valid, since, in general, they are less biased than observational studies; likewise, prospective studies are generally thought to be more reliable, since they are less biased than case-control or uncontrolled studies in terms of assessing exposure (Bush, 1990).

The major advantage of experimental studies, or clinical trials, is that they involve an unbiased assignment to treatment, allowing one to be reasonably confident that any differences in risk seen between treated and untreated women are the result of the treatment *per se*, and not other factors such as access to medical care or healthier women being selected to receive oestrogen (Bush, 1990). This is not the case in observational studies where there may be self and/or physician selection in oestrogen use.

Issues which must be taken into account when evaluating case-control studies are the representativeness of the controls compared with the general population (community controls are more representative than hospital controls), and the accuracy of information regarding exposures which may have occurred in the distant past. Issues of concern in prospective studies are

Table 1. Summary of study designs used to assess the association between oestrogen use and CVD in women.

Study design	Comments
Experimental (clinical trial)	Considered the most rigorous design; the results from clinical trials are accorded much weight. The major advantage is that selection to therapy is done in an unbiased manner. The major disadvantage is cost.
Observational:	
Prospective or cohort study	Considered the best of the observational studies, since oestrogen users and non-users are followed through time until a CVD event takes place or the study ends. The major advantage is that oestrogen use or non-use is known prior to the event. The major disadvantages are cost and the potential for biased selection to treatment.
Case-control	A useful design for studying rare diseases. The history of oestrogen use in women who have had a cardiovascular event (cases) is compared with the history in women free from disease (controls). The major advantage is low cost. The major disadvantages are differential recall of exposure between cases and controls, and the possibility that the controls are not representative of the 'healthy' population. Case-control studies which use community controls rather than hospital controls are given greater weight.
Population control	The experience of a group of oestrogen users is compared with the experience of a general population group. For example, CVD mortality in women in one large clinical practice in California is compared with CVD mortality in all women in California. The major advantage is the low cost. The major disadvantage is that the 'control' group may not be comparable to the clinic population.

those which relate to the possibility of selection to the particular treatment of interest (i.e. oestrogen use) and the concern that outcomes may be determined by factors which led to selection for treatment, and not by the treatment itself. Keeping this general framework in mind, a brief review of the published literature regarding oestrogen use and CVD in women is given below.

Experimental studies

There has been only one published clinical trial (Nachtigall et al, 1979) which has evaluated the association of oestrogen use and the risk of CVD in women (Table 2). This small trial in long-term residents of a chronic disease hospital demonstrated that those assigned to oestrogen/progestin therapy had a marked (~70%) but non-significant reduction in myocardial infarction during the 10 years of follow-up. The results from this trial have had limited impact on the assessment of the oestrogen-CVD association because they were not statistically significant and because of the selective characteristics of the participants.

Table 2. Summary of experimental studies of oestrogen use and CVD in women.

Study	Population	Follow-up	Endpoints	Risk estimate*
Nachtigall et al, 1979	168 residents of a chronic disease hospital	10 years	Fatal and non-fatal MI	0.33 (0.01–3.6)†

MI = myocardial infarction.
* Risk estimates and 95% confidence intervals either provided by the authors or calculated from available data.
† 95% confidence interval.

Prospective studies

In contrast to the one clinical trial, there have been at least 14 prospective studies which have addressed the effects of non-contraceptive oestrogen on cardiovascular risk (Table 3). These studies range in size from very small (164 women; Lafferty and Helmuth, 1985) to very large (32 000 women; Stampfer et al, 1985), and assessed a wide range of cardiovascular endpoints. In general, all had a sufficient length of follow-up (5 or more years).

Of these 14 studies, seven found statistically significant reductions of approximately 40% or more in CVD occurrence, and three found non-significant reductions of 30% or more among oestrogen users. Three additional studies found non-significant reductions in risk between 10 and 30%. Only one prospective report from the Framingham Heart Study found a significant increase in the risk of CVD among oestrogen users (Wilson et al, 1985). This finding stands in contrast to the report from Eaker and Castelli (1987), also from the Framingham Study, which found a slightly lower risk of CVD ($\sim 10\%$) among oestrogen users.

It is difficult to determine why these results from Framingham conflict with each other and with most other prospective studies. These differences between the two reports may have occurred because different endpoints were assessed, or because different analytical approaches were taken. The results may differ from the other prospective studies because the doses of oestrogen used by women in Framingham might have been higher than those used in other studies, leading to an increase in thrombogenic disease, or because women in Framingham might have been more frequently prescribed DES or other synthetic (and thus more potent) oestrogens. Another possibility is that the results occurred by chance.

Despite the divergent results from the Framingham Study, it is evident that the other prospective studies are in general agreement that oestrogen users have a markedly lower rate of CVD than non-users. In fact, 12 of the 14 studies are consistent with (e.g. their confidence limits include 0.5) the thesis that oestrogen use confers a 50% or greater reduction in CVD risk.

The major limitation of prospective studies is that it is impossible to know whether 'selection bias' to oestrogen use or oestrogen use *per se* is responsible for any observed effect. Since women who take oestrogens may be healthier than women who do not, this 'selection bias' may explain some or all of the CVD protection observed in users. 'Selection bias' can be ruled out only in randomized clinical trials; however, looking at the effects of oestrogen in selected subgroups of women, i.e. those with and without CVD, may be helpful.

In this regard, one of these prospective studies is a follow-up of women who had previously undergone angiography (Sullivan et al, 1990). In this report, all women with severe coronary stenosis (oestrogen users and non-users) were followed until death or for up to 10 years. The results of this study showed that those women with documented stenosis who used oestrogens, compared with those with documented stenosis not using them, had a significantly better overall survival (97% and 60%, respectively). Given

Table 3. Summary of prospective studies of oestrogen use and CVD in women.

Study	Population	Follow-up	Endpoint(s)	Risk estimate*
Hammond et al, 1979	301 users and 309 non-users	5.0 years	Fatal and non-fatal CVD	0.5 (0.47–0.63)†
Lafferty and Helmuth, 1985	61 users and 63 non-users	8.6 years	Fatal and non-fatal MI	0.2 (0.02–1.4)
Stampfer et al, 1985	32 317 users and non-users	4.0 years	Fatal CHD and non-fatal MI	0.3 (0.2–0.6)
Wilson et al, 1985	1234 users and non-users	?	Fatal and non-fatal CHD	1.8 ($P<0.01$)
Bush et al, 1987	593 users and 1677 non-users	8.5 years	Fatal CVD	0.3 (0.12–0.81)
Eaker and Castelli, 1987	1661 users and non-users	10 years	Fatal and non-fatal CHD	0.9 (0.47–1.6)
Petitti et al, 1987	2656 users and 3437 non-users	13 years	CVD death	0.9 (0.2–3.3)
Criqui et al, 1988	734 users and 1134 non-users	12 years	CVD death	0.8 (0.61–1.1)
Henderson et al, 1988a	8841 users and non-users	6 years	Fatal MI	0.6 (0.42–0.82)
Paganini-Hill et al, 1988	4962 users and 3845 non-users	6 years	Fatal stroke	0.5 (0.42–0.82)
Avila et al, 1990	24 900 users and non-users	6 years	Fatal and non-fatal MI	0.7 (0.3–1.3)
Sullivan et al, 1990	2268 users and non-users	10 years	Death	0.2 (0.04–0.66)
Van Der Giezen et al, 1990	13 083 users and non-users	10 years	CVD death	0.6 (0.30–1.1)
Wolf et al, 1991	1944 users and non-users	10 years	CVD death	0.7 (0.48–0.90)

MI = myocardial infarction; CHD = coronary heart disease.
* Risk estimates and 95% confidence intervals either provided by the authors or calculated from available data.
† 95% confidence interval.

these findings, it is difficult to see how selection bias could have produced these results.

Case-control studies

There have been 13 published case-control reports (Table 4) which have assessed the oestrogen-CVD association. Again, these studies range in size from very small (nine cases; Croft and Hannaford, 1989) to very large (1444 cases; Sullivan et al, 1988). Most have utilized a clinical definition of CVD, e.g. non-fatal or fatal myocardial infarction, although three (Gruchow et al, 1988; Sullivan et al, 1988; McFarland et al, 1989) utilized the degree of coronary occlusion as they were conducted in women who underwent coronary angiography.

Of these 13 studies, nine show reductions in CVD of 40% or more. Four of these estimates are statistically significant. One (Rosenberg et al, 1980) found no effect of oestrogen on CVD risk, two (La Vecchia et al, 1987; Thompson et al, 1989) found non-significant 10 to 30% increases, and one (Jick et al, 1978) found a significant 840% increased CVD risk in women using oestrogen.

It is apparent that the report from Jick et al (1978) is out of line with the other estimates. This particular study suffers from serious methodological flaws. Furthermore, it should be noted that there were only 17 cases, 16 of whom smoked, and all the women were under 45 years of age. The other two reports which show a modest but non-significant increase in CVD among users are studies with clinically defined cases from Italy (La Vecchia et al, 1987) and Great Britain (Thompson et al, 1989).

The results from these two studies are somewhat in contrast to the other studies which used clinically defined cases and found protection against CVD for users (Rosenberg et al, 1976; Talbott et al, 1977; Adam et al, 1981; Szklo et al, 1984; Beard et al, 1989; Croft and Hannaford, 1989). These latter studies report a modest (relative risk of 0.8) to substantial (relative risk of 0.3) reduction in CVD risk among oestrogen users.

It is interesting to note that all three angiography studies show significant reductions of 50 and 60% in the amount of coronary stenosis found in oestrogen users. Theoretically, studies with angiographically defined disease should provide more precise estimates of risk than studies with clinically defined endpoints. This is because misclassification of disease status is less likely to occur when the arteries are actually visualized. Given that subclinical CVD is likely to be prevalent in postmenopausal women, the reliance of a clinical definition of disease in case-control (and prospective) studies may result in estimates that are conservative or biased toward the null. This is because the 'non-diseased' group is likely to include those with subclinical CVD, leading to a diminished ability of the study to find an effect.

Again, with the notable exception of Jick et al (1978), the majority of the case-control studies report that CVD occurrence in oestrogen users is lower than in non-users. Nine of these 13 case-control reports are consistent with oestrogen use conferring a 50% or greater reduction in CVD risk, and 11 of

Table 4. Summary of case-control studies of oestrogen use and CVD in women.

Study	Population	Age (years)	Controls	Endpoint(s)	Risk estimate*
Rosenberg et al, 1976	336 cases and 6730 controls	40–75	Hospital	Non-fatal MI	0.5 (0.22–0.99)†
Talbott et al, 1977	64 cases and 64 controls	25–64	Community	Sudden death	0.3 (0.07–1.5)
Jick et al, 1978	17 cases and 34 controls	39–45	Hospital	Non-fatal MI	8.4 (1.7–45)
Rosenberg et al, 1980	477 cases and 1832 controls	30–49	Hospital	Non-fatal MI	1.0 (0.60–1.7)
Adam et al, 1981	76 cases and 151 controls	50–59	Community	Fatal MI	0.7 (0.26–1.6)
Szklo et al, 1984	39 cases and 45 controls	35–64	Hospital	Non-fatal MI	0.6 (0.20–1.9)
La Vecchia et al, 1987	116 cases and 160 controls	45–54	Hospital	Non-fatal MI	1.3 (0.55–3.1)
Gruchow et al, 1988	154 users and 779 non-users	50–75	Angiographic	Coronary occlusion	0.4 (0.29–0.46)
Sullivan et al, 1988	1444 cases and 744 controls	$\bar{x}=62.8$	Angiographic	Coronary occlusion	0.4 (0.29–0.67)
Beard et al, 1989	86 cases and 150 controls	40–59	Community	Fatal and non-fatal CHD	0.6 (0.24–1.3)
Croft and Hannaford, 1989	9 cases and 32 controls	$\bar{x}=48.4$	Physician records	Fatal and non-fatal MI	0.8 (0.3–1.8)
McFarland et al, 1989	137 cases and 208 controls	35–59	Angiographic	Coronary occlusion	0.5 (0.3–0.8)
Thompson et al, 1989	603 cases and 1206 controls	45–69	Physician records	Fatal and non-fatal MI and stroke	1.1 (0.79–1.6)

MI = myocardial infarction; CHD = coronary heart disease.
* Risk estimates and 95% confidence intervals either provided by the authors or calculated from available data.
† 95% confidence interval.

the 13 are consistent with a 30% or greater reduction in risk of the major cause of morbidity and mortality in postmenopausal women.

Population-controlled studies

The risk estimates from the three population-controlled studies are presented in Table 5. Two of the reports (Burch et al, 1974; MacMahon, 1978) are from populations identified in the United States, and the third (Hunt et al, 1987) is from Great Britain. Each of these studies found that CVD rates were significantly lower among cohorts of women using oestrogen compared with a general population of women. The risk reductions seen in the users ranged from 50 to 70%.

As noted previously, risk estimates from population-controlled studies are generally given less weight than estimates from internally controlled studies, since there is no assurance that the control population is comparable to the cohort of interest. For example, oestrogen users may have fewer CVD risk factors than women in the general population. Nonetheless, these three studies, taken together, provide additional evidence that oestrogen users are at lower risk for CVD than non-users.

Summary

The clear majority of studies which examined the effect of non-contraceptive oestrogen on CVD found moderate to marked reductions in CVD among users. In fact, of the 31 studies evaluated (one clinical trial, 14 prospective, 13 case-control and three population-controlled), 28 are consistent with a 30% or greater reduction in the risk of CVD among users, and 25 are consistent with a 50% or greater risk reduction. A meta-analysis of these 31 reports, weighting each risk estimate for size and type of study, finds an overall relative risk of 0.45. Clearly, at this time, the evidence strongly supports the contention that unopposed oestrogen use is associated with a marked reduction in CVD occurrence.

Unfortunately, only three of these studies address the effect of oestrogen/progestin use on cardiovascular risk (Nachtigall et al, 1979; Hunt et al, 1987; Thompson et al, 1989). The study by Nachtigall et al (1979) was very small, but the results were reassuring, as women assigned to the oestrogen/progestin therapy had a marked reduction in CVD occurrence. The other two studies (Hunt et al, 1987; Thompson et al, 1989) were conducted in Great Britain and, like the clinical trial, are limited by small numbers of users and various progestin formulations and dosages. However, these reports are also generally reassuring in that risk estimates for CVD among oestrogen/progestin users were not elevated. In the population-controlled study by Hunt et al (1987), use of oestrogen and progestin was associated with a moderate (relative risk of 0.5) reduction in CVD occurrence, while Thompson et al (1989) found a more moderate (relative risk of 0.8) reduction in risk.

Thompson et al (1989) also evaluated the effect of progestin only on

Table 5. Summary of population-control studies of oestrogen use and CVD in women.

Study	Comparison	Follow-up	Endpoint(s)	Risk estimate*
Burch et al, 1974	737 users/unknown	13.3 years	CHD deaths	0.4
MacMahon, 1978	1891 users/US women	12.0 years	ASHD deaths	0.3
Hunt et al, 1987	4544 users/English and Welsh women	5.6 years	CVD deaths	0.5

CHD = coronary heart disease; ASHD = arteriosclerotic heart disease.
* Risk estimates are all statistically significant.

CVD, and found that unopposed progestin use was associated with a significantly elevated risk of CVD (relative risk of 1.9; confidence limit (CL) = 1.1–3.2). One concern, given these three studies, is that the effect of progestin on CVD risk may diminish or cancel the beneficial effects of unopposed oestrogen. Clearly, while the studies are in general agreement that unopposed oestrogen is beneficial, additional studies of oestrogen/ progestin therapy and CVD risk are needed. Given the problems of selection bias inherent in observational studies, a clinical trial of oestrogen and oestrogen/progestin therapy is necessary.

CONTROVERSY IN THE OESTROGEN-CVD ASSOCIATION

Parenteral oestrogen therapy

As noted earlier, the marked first-pass hepatic metabolism of orally administered oestrogens is thought to be responsible for many of the deleterious side-effects of oestrogen therapy (Cedars and Judd, 1987). However, it is this same first-pass phenomenon that is thought to be responsible, at least in part, for the cardioprotective effects of oestrogen therapy, presumably through favourable alterations in hepatic lipoprotein biosynthesis and metabolism (Cedars and Judd, 1987; Bush et al, 1987; Burkman, 1988; Miller-Bass and Adashi, 1990). Beneficial changes in the lipoprotein profile—increases in high density lipoprotein (HDL), the protective lipoprotein fraction, and decreases in low density lipoprotein (LDL), the atherogenic lipoprotein fraction—seen during oestrogen therapy have been well documented (Hazzard, 1989; Lobo, 1990). It is estimated that 25 to 50% of the cardioprotective effects of oestrogen therapy are mediated through these favourable changes in the lipoprotein profile (Bush et al, 1987; Gruchow et al, 1988). Thus, while parenteral routes of oestrogen therapy might be expected to reduce the incidence of unwanted side-effects through limited first-pass metabolism, they might also be assumed to provide little in the way of cardioprotection. However, there is evidence that lipoprotein levels may be beneficially altered with parenteral oestrogen therapy.

Both intramuscular oestrogen and oestrogen delivered via subdermal pellets have been shown to elevate HDL levels. At least two studies have demonstrated a significant increase in HDL levels following a single 10 mg injection of 17β-oestradiol valerate or 17β-oestradiol phenylpropionate plus 17β-oestradiol benzoate (Punnonen and Rauramo, 1980; Sherwin et al, 1987) with concomitant, but transient, decreases in LDL as well (Sherwin et al, 1987). Similarly, several investigators have documented significant increases in HDL levels following the insertion of subdermal pellets containing 25–100 mg of 17β-oestradiol (Lobo et al, 1980; Farish et al, 1984; Sharf et al, 1985; Stanczyk et al, 1988). However, such pellets appear to have little, if any, effect on LDL levels (Lobo, 1980; Farish et al, 1984; Stanczyk et al, 1988).

Initial studies involving the use of transdermal and percutaneous 17β-oestradiol preparations seemed to indicate that, as expected, their lack of significant first-class metabolism would result in little change in the serum lipid profiles of patients receiving these forms of oestrogen therapy. Short-term (4–8 weeks) use of standard doses of both transdermal and per-cutaneous 17β-oestradiol resulted in no change in either HDL or LDL levels (Chetkowski et al, 1986; De Lignieres et al, 1986; Haas et al, 1988). However, subsequent studies involving long-term use of both preparations have documented many of the same beneficial lipid changes noted in patients receiving oral oestrogen therapy (Jensen et al, 1987; Stanczyk et al, 1988). Significant increases in HDL levels have been reported in patients following use of transdermal 17β-oestradiol (0.10 mg/dl) for 24 weeks (Stanczyk et al, 1988). In a 2-year placebo-controlled trial, Jensen et al (1987) observed significant decreases in both LDL and total cholesterol levels in patients using percutaneous 17β-oestradiol (3 mg/dl) at the end of the first year. Significant increases in HDL levels were noted by the end of the second year. It appears that long-term use of these preparations is necessary to achieve favourable changes in lipid profiles.

While the cardioprotective effects of oestrogen therapy can be explained, in part, by the favourable effects of oestrogen on lipids, there is also evidence that oestrogen has direct effects on the cardiovascular system. Studies in animals, including non-human primates, have documented the presence of oestrogen receptors in both the myocardium and aorta, and have demonstrated that these are physiologically functional (McGill, 1989). Clearly, parenteral oestrogen therapy would be as effective as oral oestrogen therapy in interacting with these receptors, and perhaps even more so when delivered directly into the bloodstream.

Effects of progestins

Synthetic progestins have effects on lipoproteins that are in direct opposition to those of oestrogen therapy: i.e. HDL levels are decreased, while LDL levels are increased (Notelovitz, 1989). This fact has created considerable concern over the use of progestin therapy in combination with oestrogen therapy. On the one hand, progestins are necessary to prevent an increased risk of endometrial cancer in women with an intact uterus who are receiving oestrogen therapy. On the other, the addition of progestins to an oestrogen therapy regimen may negate or even overwhelm the beneficial effects of oestrogen therapy on cardiovascular risk.

While there are few long-term studies evaluating the effects of progestin addition to oestrogen therapy on the risk of CVD, there are some studies documenting the effects of added progestins on the lipid changes seen with oestrogen therapy. While some investigators have reported reversal of favourable lipid patterns in oestrogen therapy users following the addition of sequential progestins (Mishell, 1989; Whitehead et al, 1990), others have documented no alteration in the beneficial effects of oestrogen therapy when progestins were added to the regimen for up to 12 days each month (Jensen et al, 1987; Kable et al, 1990).

More recently, studies involving the use of small continuous daily doses of a progestin (2.5 mg medroxyprogesterone acetate) in combination with daily oestrogen administration have, in general, reported changes in lipids that appear to be favourable (Whitehead et al, 1990). However, these studies suffer from a number of flaws in both design and methodology, most notably the lack of an untreated control group in many instances (Whitehead et al, 1990). The use of continuous combined oestrogen/ progestin regimens is the subject of an extensive review by Whitehead et al (1990) and the reader is referred to this for more detailed information. It is obvious that the questions concerning the effects of progestin administration on the cardioprotection afforded by oestrogen therapy are far from being answered, and prudence dictates that progestins be used only in women with intact uteri and in the smallest possible dose which will still provide endometrial protection (Lobo, 1990). Again, the PEPI trial underway in the United States will provide more definitive answers within a few years.

CONCLUSION

Oestrogen therapy offers a number of advantages to menopausal and postmenopausal women. It relieves menopausal symptoms, provides protection from osteoporosis and, as is becoming increasingly clear, provides protection from CVD as well. A review of the medical literature supports the thesis that oestrogen therapy is associated with a 50% decrease in the risk of CVD in women. Some, but probably not all, of the benefit of oestrogen on CVD risk is mediated through changes in lipoproteins, specifically increases in HDL cholesterol.

Risks of oestrogen therapy include an increase in endometrial cancer. Although there is the possibility of an increased risk of hypertension, hypercoagulability and gallbladder disease in oestrogen users due to the 'first-pass' effect, there is little evidence to suggest that these conditions are increased in users. Furthermore, while some suggest that long-term oestrogen use is associated with an increase in breast cancer, clear and compelling evidence linking oestrogen use to breast cancer occurrence is not yet evident.

Recent studies involving the long-term use of parenteral oestrogens suggest that these alternate forms of oestrogen therapy may provide cardioprotection that is similar to that seen with traditional oral oestrogen therapy, although follow-up studies of cardiovascular morbidity and mortality will be necessary to provide conclusive evidence.

While the addition of a progestational agent to oestrogen therapy protects against an increased risk of endometrial cancer, it may reverse the beneficial lipid changes induced by unopposed oestrogen. Additionally, little is known regarding the effect of progestational agents on the risk of breast cancer. Given the large potential benefit of oestrogen use (e.g. significant reductions in CVD) and the lack of evidence on progestin use, well-designed studies and/or trials to address the question of oestrogen and oestrogen/progestin effects on disease outcomes, particularly CVD, are urgently needed.

REFERENCES

Adam S, Williams V & Vessey MP (1981) Cardiovascular disease and hormone replacement treatment: a pilot case-control study. *British Medical Journal* **282**: 1277–1278.

Avila MH, Walker AM & Jick H (1990) Use of replacement estrogens and the risk of myocardial infarction. *Epidemiology* **1**: 128–133.

Barrett-Connor E (1990) Putative complications of estrogen replacement therapy: hypertension, diabetes, thrombophlebitis and gallstones. In Korman SG (ed.) *The Menopause: Biological and Clinical Consequences of Ovarian Failure: Evolution and Management*, pp 199–210. Massachusetts: Serono Symposia.

Beard CM, Kottke TE, Annegers JF & Ballard DJ (1989) The Rochester Coronary Heart Disease Project: effect of cigarette smoking, hypertension, diabetes, and steroidal estrogen use on coronary heart disease among 40- to 59-year-old women, 1960 through 1982. *Mayo Clinic Proceedings* **64**: 1471–1480.

Bergkvist L, Adami H-O, Persson I et al (1989a) The risk of breast cancer after estrogen and estrogen-progestin replacement. *New England Journal of Medicine* **321**: 293–297.

Bergkvist L, Adami H-O, Persson I et al (1989a) Prognosis after cancer diagnosis in women exposed to estrogen and estrogen-progestogen replacement therapy. *American Journal of Epidemiology* **130**: 221–228.

Boston Collaborative Drug Surveillance Program (1974) Surgically confirmed gallbladder disease, venous thromboembolism, and breast tumors in relation to postmenopausal estrogen therapy. *New England Journal of Medicine* **290**: 15–19.

Burch JC, Byrd BF Jr & Vaughn WK (1974) The effects of long-term estrogen on hysterectomized women. *American Journal of Obstetrics and Gynecology* **118**: 778–782.

Burkman RT (1988) Lipid and lipoprotein changes in relation to oral contraception and hormonal replacement therapy. *Fertility and Sterility* **49(supplement)**: 39s–50s.

Bush TL (1990) Noncontraceptive estrogen use and risk of cardiovascular disease: an overview and critique of the literature. In Korman SG (ed.) *The Menopause: Biological and Clinical Consequences of Ovarian Failure: Evolution and Management*, pp 211–224. Massachusetts: Serono Symposia.

Bush TL & Barrett-Connor E (1985) Noncontraceptive estrogen use and cardiovascular disease. *Epidemiologic Reviews* **7**: 80–104.

Bush TL, Cowan LD, Barrett-Connor E et al (1983) Estrogen use and all-cause mortality. *Journal of the American Medical Association* **249**: 903–906.

Bush TL, Barrett-Connor E, Cowan LD et al (1987) Cardiovascular mortality and noncontraceptive use of estrogen in women. *Circulation* **75**: 1102–1109.

Callantine MR, Martin PL, Bolding OT et al (1975) Micronized 17-β estradiol for oral estrogen therapy in menopausal women. *Obstetrics and Gynecology* **46**: 37–41.

Campbell S & Whitehead M (1977) Oestrogen therapy and the menopausal syndrome. *Clinics in Obstetrics and Gynaecology* **4**: 31–47.

Cedars MI & Judd HL (1987) Nonoral routes of estrogen administration. *Obstetrics and Gynecology Clinics of North America* **14**: 269–298.

Chetkowski RJ, Meldrum DR, Steingold KA et al (1986) Biologic effects of transdermal estradiol. *New England Journal of Medicine* **314**: 1615–1620.

Colditz GA, Stampfer MJ, Willett WC et al (1990) Prospective study of estrogen replacement therapy and risk of breast cancer in postmenopausal women. *Journal of the American Medical Association* **264**: 2648–2653.

Collins J, Donner A, Allen LH et al (1980) Oestrogen use and survival in endometrial cancer. *Lancet* **ii**: 961–964.

Coope J, Thompson JM & Poller L (1975) Effects of 'natural oestrogen' replacement therapy on menopausal symptoms and blood clotting. *British Medical Journal* **284**: 139–143.

Criqui MH, Suarez L, Barrett-Connor E et al (1988) Postmenopausal estrogen use and mortality. Results from a prospective study in a defined homogeneous community. *American Journal of Epidemiology* **128**: 606–614.

Croft P & Hannaford PC (1989) Risk factors for acute myocardial infarction in women: evidence from the Royal College of General Practitioners' oral contraception study. *British Medical Journal* **298**: 165–168.

De Lignieres B, Basdevant A, Thomas G et al (1986) Biological effects of estradiol-17β in postmenopausal women: oral versus percutaneous administration. *Journal of Clinical Endocrinology and Metabolism* **62**: 536–541.

Dupont WD & Page DL (1991) Menopausal estrogen replacement therapy and breast cancer. *Archives of Internal Medicine* **151**: 67–72.

Eaker E & Castelli W (1987) Coronary heart disease and its risk factors among women in the Framingham Study. In Eaker E, Packard B, Wenger N et al (eds) *Coronary Heart Disease in Women*, pp 122–130. New York: Haymarket Doyma.

Farish E, Fletcher CD, Hart DM et al (1984) The effects of hormone implants on serum lipoproteins and steroid hormones in bilaterally oophorectomized women. *Acta Endocrinologica* **106**: 116–120.

Fried LP, Bush TL & Whelton PT (1987) Attributable risk of morbidity: a method for assessing disease impact in the elderly. *American Journal of Epidemiology* **126**: 489(abstract).

Gambrell RD (1990) Prognosis after breast cancer diagnosis in women exposed to estrogen and estrogen-progestogen replacement therapy. *American Journal of Epidemiology* **132**: 1017(letter).

Genant HK, Baylink DJ & Gallagher JC (1989) Estrogens in the prevention of osteoporosis in postmenopausal women. *American Journal of Obstetrics and Gynecology* **161**: 1842–1846.

Geola FL, Frumar AM, Tataryn IV et al (1980) Biological effects of various doses of conjugated equine estrogens in postmenopausal women. *Journal of Clinical Endocrinology and Metabolism* **51**: 620–625.

Goebelsmann U, Mashchak CA & Mishell DR (1985) Comparison of hepatic impact of oral and vaginal administration of ethinyl estradiol. *American Journal of Obstetrics and Gynecology* **151**: 868–877.

Gordon GB, Bush TL, Helzlsouer KJ et al (1990) Relationship of serum levels of dehydroepiandrosterone and dehydroepiandrosterone sulfate to the risk of developing postmenopausal breast cancer. *Cancer Research* **50**: 3859–3862.

Gruchow HW, Anderson AJ, Barboriak JJ et al (1988) Postmenopausal use of estrogen and occlusion of coronary arteries. *American Heart Journal* **115**: 954–963.

Haas S, Walsh B, Evans S et al (1988) The effect of transdermal estradiol on hormone and metabolic dynamics over a six-week period. *Obstetrics and Gynecology* **71**: 671–676.

Hammond CB, Jelovsek FR, Lee KL et al (1979) Effect of long-term estrogen replacement therapy. I. Metabolic effects. *American Journal of Obstetrics and Gynecology* **133**: 525–536.

Harris RB, Laws A, Reddy VM et al (1990) Are women using postmenopausal estrogens? A community survey. *American Journal of Public Health* **80**: 1266–1268.

Havlik RJ, Liu BM, Kovar MG et al (1987) Health statistics on older persons, United States, 1986. *Vital and Health Statistics*, series 3, no. 25 (DHHS publication no. (PHS) 87–1409). Washington, DC: US Government Printing Office.

Hazzard WR (1989) Estrogen replacement and cardiovascular disease: serum lipids and blood pressure effects. *American Journal of Obstetrics and Gynecology* **161**: 1847–1853.

Hemminki E, Kennedy DL, Baum C et al (1988) Prescribing of non-contraceptive estrogens and progestins in the United States, 1974–86. *American Journal of Public Health* **78**: 1479–1481.

Henderson BE (1989) The cancer question: an overview of recent epidemiologic and retrospective data. *American Journal of Obstetrics and Gynecology* **161**: 1859–1864.

Henderson BE, Paganini-Hill A & Ross RK (1988a) Estrogen replacement therapy and protection from acute myocardial infarction. *American Journal of Obstetrics and Gynecology* **159**: 312–317.

Henderson BE, Ross R & Bernstein L (1988b) Estrogens as a cause of human cancer: The Richard and Hinda Rosenthal Foundation Award Lecture. *Cancer Research* **48**: 246–253.

Henderson BE, Paganini-Hill A & Ross R (1991) Decreased mortality in users of estrogen replacement therapy. *Archives of Internal Medicine* **151**: 75–78.

Holst J, Cajander S, Carlstrom K et al (1983) Percutaneous estrogen replacement therapy: effects on circulating estrogens, gonadotropins and prolactin. *Acta Obstetrica et Gynecologica Scandinavica* **62**: 49–53.

Hulka BS, Kaufman DG, Fowler WC et al (1980) Predominance of early endometrial cancers after long-term estrogen use. *Journal of the American Medical Association* **244**: 2419–2422.

Hunt K, Vessey M, McPherson K et al (1987) Long-term surveillance of mortality and cancer incidence in women receiving hormone replacement therapy. *British Journal of Obstetrics and Gynaecology* **94:** 620–635.

Jensen J, Riis BJ, Strom V et al (1987) Long-term effects of percutaneous estrogens and oral progesterone on serum lipoproteins in postmenopausal women. *American Journal of Obstetrics and Gynecology* **156:** 66–71.

Jick H, Dinan B & Rothman KJ (1978) Noncontraceptive estrogens and nonfatal myocardial infarction. *Journal of the American Medical Association* **239:** 1407–1409.

Judd HL, Meldrum DR, Deftos LJ et al (1983) Estrogen replacement therapy: indications and complications. *Annals of Internal Medicine* **98:** 195–205.

Kable WT, Gallagher JC, Nachtigall L et al (1990) Lipid changes after hormone replacement therapy for menopause. *Journal of Reproductive Medicine* **35:** 513–518.

Lafferty FW & Helmuth DO (1985) Post-menopausal estrogen replacement: the prevention of osteoporosis and systemic effects. *Maturitas* **7:** 147–159.

Laufer LR, De Fazio JL, Lu JKH et al (1983) Estrogen replacement therapy by trans-dermal estradiol administration. *American Journal of Obstetrics and Gynecology* **146:** 533–538.

La Vecchia C, Franceshi S, Decarli AS et al (1987) Risk factors for myocardial infarction in young women. *American Journal of Epidemiology* **125:** 832–843.

Liang AP, Levenson AG, Layde PM et al (1983) Risk of breast, uterine corpus, and ovarian cancer in women receiving medroxyprogesterone injections. *Journal of the American Medical Association* **249:** 2909–2912.

Lipsett MB (1986) Steroids and carcinogenesis. In Gregoire AT & Blye RT (eds) *Contraceptive Steroids: Pharmacology and Safety*, pp 215–229. New York: Plenum.

Lobo RA (1989) Cardiovascular disease, menopause, and the influence of hormone replacement therapy. *Progress in Clinical and Biological Research* **320:** 313–332.

Lobo RA (1990) Cardiovascular implications of estrogen replacement therapy. *Obstetrics and Gynecology* **75(supplement):** 18s–25s.

Lobo RA, March CM, Goebelsmann U et al (1980) Subdermal estradiol pellets following hysterectomy and oophorectomy: effect upon serum estrone, estradiol, luteinizing hormone, follicle stimulating hormone, corticosteroid binding globulin-binding capacity, lipids, and hot flushes. *American Journal of Obstetrics and Gynecology* **138:** 714–719.

Luotola H (1983) Blood pressure and hemodynamics in postmenopausal women during estradiol-17β substitution. *Annals of Clinical Research* **15(supplement 38):** 1–121.

MacMahon B (1978) Cardiovascular disease and non-contraceptive oestrogen therapy. In Oliver MF (ed.) *Coronary Heart Disease in Young Women*, pp 197–202. Edinburgh: Churchill Livingstone.

Mandel FP, Geola FL, Lu JKH et al (1982) Biologic effects of various doses of ethinyl estradiol in postmenopausal women. *Obstetrics and Gynecology* **59:** 673–679.

Mandel FP, Geola FL, Meldrum DR et al (1983) Biological effects of various doses of vaginally administered conjugated equine estrogens in postmenopausal women. *Journal of Clinical Endocrinology and Metabolism* **57:** 133–139.

Martin PL, Burnier AM & Greaney MO (1972) Oral menopausal therapy using 17-β micronized estradiol. *Obstetrics and Gynecology* **39:** 771–774.

Mashchak CA, Lobo RA, Dozono-Takano R et al (1982) Comparison of pharmacodynamic properties of various estrogen formulations. *American Journal of Obstetrics and Gynecology* **144:** 511–518.

McFarland KF, Boniface ME, Hornung CA et al (1989) Risk factors and noncontraceptive estrogen use in women with and without coronary disease. *American Heart Journal* **117:** 1209–1214.

McGill HC (1989) Sex steroid hormone receptors in the cardiovascular system. *Postgraduate Medicine* **Apr:** 64–68.

Miller-Bass K & Adashi EY (1990) Current status and future prospects of transdermal estrogen replacement therapy. *Fertility and Sterility* **53:** 961–974.

Mishell DR (1989) Use of progestins. *Postgraduate Medicine* **Apr:** 84–88.

Nachtigall LE, Nachtigall RH, Nachtigall RD et al (1979) Estrogen replacement therapy. II. A prospective study in the relationship to carcinoma and cardiovascular and metabolic problems. *Obstetrics and Gynecology* **54:** 74–79.

National Center for Health Statistics (1986) Moss AJ, Parsons VL. Current estimates from National Health Interview Survey, United States, 1985. *Vital and Health Statistics*, series

10, no. 160 (DHHS publication no. 86–1588). Washington, DC: US Government Printing Office.

National Center for Health Statistics (1990) *Vital Statistics of the United States*, 1987, vol. II: Mortality, part A (DHHS publication no. 90–1101, Public Health Service). Washington, DC: US Government Printing Office.

Notelovitz M (1989) Estrogen replacement therapy: indications, contraindications, and agent selection. *American Journal of Obstetrics and Gynecology* **161:** 1832–1841.

Padwick ML, Endacott J & Whitehead MI (1985) Efficacy, acceptability, and metabolic effects of transdermal estradiol in the management of postmenopausal women. *American Journal of Obstetrics and Gynecology* **152:** 1085–1091.

Paganini-Hill A, Ross RK & Henderson BE (1988) Postmenopausal oestrogen treatment and stroke: a prospective study. *British Medical Journal* **297:** 519–522.

Persson I, Adami HO, Bergkvist L et al (1989) Risk of endometrial cancer after treatment with oestrogens alone or in conjunction with progestogens: results of a prospective study. *British Medical Journal* **298:** 147–151.

Persson I, Adami HO & Bergkvist L (1990) Hormone replacement therapy and the risk of cancer in the breast and reproductive organs: a review of epidemiological data. In Drife JO & Studd JWW (eds) *HRT and Osteoporosis*, pp 165–175. London: Springer-Verlag.

Petitti DB, Perlman JA & Sidney S (1987) Noncontraceptive estrogens and mortality: long-term follow-up of women in the Walnut Creek Study. *Obstetrics and Gynecology* **70:** 289–293.

Porter LE, Van Thiel DH & Eagon PK (1987) Estrogens and progestins as tumor inducers. *Seminars in Liver Disease* **7:** 24–31.

Punnonen R & Rauramo L (1980) The effect of castration and estrogen therapy on serum high-density lipoprotein cholesterol. *International Journal of Gynaecology and Obstetrics* **17:** 434–436.

Ravnikar V (1990) Physiology and treatment of hot flushes. *Obstetrics and Gynecology* **75(supplement):** 3s–8s.

Rosenberg A, Armstrong B, Jick H et al (1976) Myocardial infarction and estrogen therapy in postmenopausal women. *New England Journal of Medicine* **294:** 1256–1259.

Rosenberg L, Slone D, Shapiro S et al (1980) Noncontraceptive estrogens and myocardial infarction in young women. *Journal of the American Medical Association* **244:** 339–342.

Selby, PI & Peacock M (1986) The effect of transdermal oestrogen on bone, calcium-regulating hormones and liver in postmenopausal women. *Clinical Endocrinology* **25:** 543–547.

Sharf M, Oettinger M, Lanir A et al (1985) Lipid and lipoprotein levels following pure estradiol implantation in post-menopausal women. *Gynecologic and Obstetric Investigation* **19:** 207–212.

Sherwin BB, Gelfand MM, Schucher R et al (1987) Postmenopausal estrogen and androgen replacement and lipoprotein lipid concentrations. *American Journal of Obstetrics and Gynecology* **156:** 414–419.

Stampfer MJ, Willett WC, Colditz GA et al (1985) A prospective study of postmenopausal estrogen therapy and coronary heart disease. *New England Journal of Medicine* **313:** 1044–1049.

Stanczyk FZ, Shoupe D, Nunez V et al (1988) A randomized comparison of nonoral estradiol delivery in postmenopausal women. *American Journal of Obstetrics and Gynecology* **159:** 1540–1546.

Stumpf PG (1990) Pharmacokinetics of estrogen. *Obstetrics and Gynecology* **75(supplement):** 9s–14s.

Sullivan JM, Vander Zwaag R, Lemp GF et al (1988) Postmenopausal estrogen use and coronary atherosclerosis. *Annals of Internal Medicine* **108:** 358–363.

Sullivan JM, Vander Zwaag R, Hughes MA et al (1990) Estrogen replacement and coronary artery disease. Effect on survival in postmenopausal women. *Archives of Internal Medicine* **150:** 2557–2562.

Szklo M, Tonascia J, Gordis L et al (1984) Estrogen use and myocardial infarction risk: a case-control study. *Preventive Medicine* **13:** 510–516.

Talbott E, Kuller LH, Detre K et al (1977) Biologic and psychosocial risk factors of sudden death from coronary disease in white women. *American Journal of Cardiology* **39:** 858–864.

Thompson SG, Meade TW & Greenberg G (1989) The use of hormonal replacement therapy and the risk of stroke and myocardial infarction in women. *Journal of Epidemiology and Community Health* **43:** 173–178.

Utian WH (1990) Current perspectives in the management of the menopausal and postmenopausal patient: introduction. *Obstetrics and Gynecology* **75(supplement):** 1s–2s.

Van Der Giezen AM, Van Kessel JGS-G, Schouten EG et al (1990) Systolic blood pressure and cardiovascular mortality among 13 740 Dutch women. *Preventive Medicine* **19:** 456–465.

Weiss NS, Lyon JL, Krishnamurthy S et al (1982) Non-contraceptive estrogen use and the occurrence of ovarian cancer. *Journal of the National Cancer Institute* **68:** 95–98.

Whitehead MI & Fraser D (1987) Controversies concerning the safety of estrogen replacement therapy. *American Journal of Obstetrics and Gynecology* **156:** 1313–1322.

Whitehead MI, Hilliard TC & Crook D (1990) The role and use of progestogens. *Obstetrics and Gynecology* **75(supplement):** 59s–76s.

Wilson PWF, Garrison RJ & Castelli WP (1985) Postmenopausal estrogen use, cigarette smoking, and cardiovascular morbidity in women over 50. *New England Journal of Medicine* **313:** 1038–1043.

Wolf PH, Madans JH, Finucane FF et al (1991) Reduction of cardiovascular disease-related mortality among postmenopausal women who use hormones: Evidence from a national cohort. *American Journal of Obstetrics and Gynecology* **164:** 489–494.

10

Effects of oestrogens and progestogens on coronary atherosclerosis and osteoporosis of monkeys

MICHAEL R. ADAMS
J. KOUDY WILLIAMS
THOMAS B. CLARKSON
MANUEL J. JAYO

THE CYNOMOLGUS MACAQUE MODEL OF MALE/FEMALE DIFFERENCES IN CORONARY ATHEROSCLEROSIS

Differences in plasma lipoproteins and coronary atherosclerosis of males and premenopausal females

Research on the pathogenesis of coronary artery atherosclerosis and coronary heart disease in females has been hampered by the lack of a suitable animal model of atherosclerosis in female human beings. Summarized in this section are data related to the development of a non-human primate model of female protection and some observations on biological and psychosocial influences on coronary artery atherosclerosis of female monkeys. Published information documenting that males of that species develop extensive main-branch coronary artery atherosclerosis when fed a cholesterol-containing diet (Clarkson et al, 1976), the existence of a menstrual cycle similar to that of female human beings (Mahoney, 1970; MacDonald, 1971; Jewett and Dukelow, 1972) and the extensive bibliography on their social behaviour (Kaplan et al, 1985) support the selection of cynomolgus monkeys as models of female protection from coronary artery atherosclerosis.

Our first experiment on male/female differences in the response of cynomolgus monkeys to a cholesterol-containing diet was focused primarily on changes in the plasma lipoproteins and on the extensiveness of coronary artery atherosclerosis. Like premenopausal women, cynomolgus macaque females had significantly higher plasma concentrations of high density lipoprotein cholesterol (HDL-C) than their male counterparts. Histological examinations of coronary arteries revealed male/female differences in the extent of coronary artery atherosclerosis (Hamm et al, 1983). Plaque extent in male and female cynomolgus macaques are presented in Figure 1 as the mean percent lumen stenosis.

Baillière's Clinical Obstetrics and Gynaecology—
Vol. 5, No. 4, December 1991
ISBN 0–7020–1548–2

915

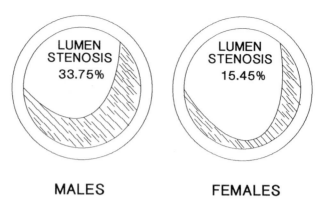

MALES   FEMALES

Figure 1. Mean coronary artery lumen stenosis of male and premenopausal female cynomolgus monkeys fed an atherogenic diet. Modified from Hamm et al (1983).

The male/female difference in coronary artery atherosclerosis among animals consuming the moderately atherogenic diet is comparable to the male/female difference in coronary artery lesion extent among New Orleans Caucasians (Tejada et al, 1968).

Effect of stress on ovarian function, plasma lipoproteins and coronary atherosclerosis

Subsequently, we considered social status (competitive dominance) and the development of coronary artery atherosclerosis among intact female cynomolgus macaques fed moderate amounts of dietary cholesterol. We found that subordinate females in social units of stable composition had more extensive coronary artery atherosclerosis than their dominant counterparts (Figure 2) (Hamm et al, 1983; Kaplan et al, 1984; Adams et al, 1985). Associated with low social status and increased coronary artery atherosclerosis were rather large decreases in plasma concentrations of HDL-C (Figure 2). In a later study we found that low social status was only associated with reduced plasma HDL-C concentrations in socially subordinate monkeys with stress-induced impairment of ovarian function (Kaplan et al, 1984).

Social subordination diminished the number of ovulatory cycles (Walker et al, 1983) and impaired reproductive success (Drickamer, 1974; Sade et al, 1976; Wilson et al, 1978; Dittus, 1979; Silk et al, 1981) among female macaques. The physiological basis seems to be that neural responses associated with psychosocial stress operate through the hypothalamopituitary axis to induce ovarian dysfunction (Bowman et al, 1978; Christian, 1980). For these reasons it was interesting to us to compare the menstrual cycles of our dominant and subordinate monkeys. We found that socially subordinate females had fewer ovulatory menstrual cycles and more cycles with deficient luteal phase progesterone concentrations than did dominant females.

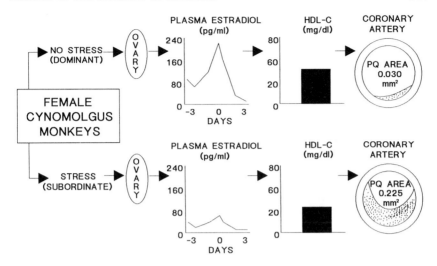

Figure 2. Stress, oestrogen deficiency, HDL-C and coronary atherosclerosis in cynomolgus macaques. PQ = plaque area. Modified from Adams et al (1985).

In that same study we noted that the luteal phase plasma progesterone concentration provided a good index of ovulatory function. Among chronically stressed subordinate females there was a strong positive correlation between mean peak plasma progesterone concentration and plasma HDL-C concentration $(r = 0.86; P < 0.001)$. This observation did not suggest to us a direct effect of endogenous progesterone on plasma HDL-C concentration, but rather a relationship between relative oestrogen deficiency and low plasma HDL-C concentrations. That conclusion is supported further by the finding that the cycles with deficient luteal phase plasma progesterone concentrations also had low periovulatory plasma oestradiol concentrations (Adams et al, 1985).

Effect of pregnancy on plasma lipoproteins and coronary atherosclerosis

Frequent pregnancy is associated with a marked reduction in the extent of coronary artery atherosclerosis (Adams et al, 1987a). This difference is probably not due to changes in total plasma cholesterol (TPC) or HDL-C concentrations. Although pregnancy resulted in dramatic decreases in both TPC and HDL-C concentrations, the fact that both were decreased meant that there was no between-group difference in the ratio of TPC to HDL-C concentrations. This ratio is a better predictor of coronary risk than either measure alone. To assess possible relationships between plasma oestradiol or progesterone concentrations and the extent of atherosclerosis, values for each were plotted and an area under the curve was calculated to use as an index of endogenous oestrogen and progesterone 'exposure' over the course of the experiment (Adams et al, 1987a). When ranked and divided into thirds of high, mid range or low plasma oestradiol index, it was found that

the coronary artery intimal area decreased with increasing plasma 17-
β-oestradiol exposure. Females in the high oestradiol group had a mean
peak plasma oestradiol of 657 pg/ml and were pregnant for an average of 15
out of the 30 months. These females were virtually unaffected by coronary
artery atherosclerosis. In contrast, females in the low oestradiol group were
pregnant an average of only 8 months and had mean peak plasma oestradiol
concentrations of 335 pg/ml. The extent of coronary artery atherosclerosis
was not different between this low oestradiol group and all non-pregnant
females. Among pregnant females, the oestradiol index was the variable
that correlated most strongly with coronary artery atherosclerosis
($r_s = -0.66$; $P < 0.01$). Also correlated with the extent of coronary artery
atherosclerosis were TPC ($r_s = -0.52$; $P < 0.01$) and HDL-C concentration
($r_s = -0.48$; $P < 0.05$). Variables that did not correlate with the extent of
coronary artery atherosclerosis were plasma progesterone, systolic blood
pressure and diastolic blood pressure.

Taken together, the results of these studies have indicated that factors
that influence endogenous sex steroid levels also influence the atherosclerotic process, and that there is a relationship between circulating oestradiol
concentrations and the extent of coronary artery atherosclerosis.

CONTRACEPTIVE STEROID EFFECTS ON PLASMA LIPOPROTEINS AND CORONARY ATHEROSCLEROSIS OF FEMALE CYNOMOLGUS MACAQUES

The inverse relationship between plasma HDL-C and the risk for coronary
heart disease has been well established for both men and women (Figure 3)
(Kannel et al, 1979).

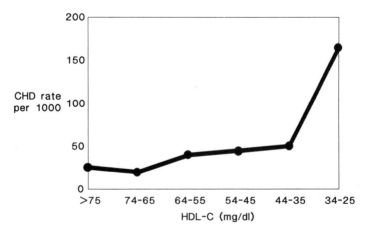

Figure 3. Coronary heart disease (CHD) and HDL-C concentrations in women ages 50 to 80
years. Modified from Kannel et al (1979).

Some steroid contraceptives reduce HDL-C in women to concentrations presumed to increase the risk of coronary heart disease (Tikkanen and Nikkila, 1986). However, there is no experimental or epidemiological evidence to support the belief that contraceptive steroid-induced decreases in HDL-C change either the extensiveness of coronary artery atherosclerosis or the risk for coronary heart disease.

The contraceptive steroid-induced dyslipoproteinaemia of female cynomolgus macaques and women is similar: modest increases in plasma low density lipoprotein (LDL) cholesterol and plasma triglyceride concentrations and decreases in HDL-C (Adams et al, 1983; Koritnik et al, 1986).

Reviewed here are the results of a large study in which we compared the effects of two contraceptive steroids on diet-induced atherosclerosis in female cynomolgus macaques (Clarkson et al, 1990). Both contained equivalent amounts of ethinyl oestradiol but structurally and pharmacologically different progestins—norgestrel (Ovral) or ethynodiol diacetate (Demulen).

In a previous study (Adams et al, 1987b) we reported a striking diminution of coronary atherosclerosis as a result of contraceptive steroid treatment among the monkeys at risk based on their plasma lipid profiles. Therefore, we analysed the data from this experiment considering all the animals, including those at high risk (TPC/HDL-C > 4.5).

The effect of the contraceptive steroid treatments on the plasma lipoprotein concentrations of all the animals and the high risk group are summarized in Figures 4 and 5, respectively.

Effects on HDL subfraction heterogeneity were also determined (Parks et al, 1989). The marked decrease in plasma HDL-C observed with two treatment groups were accounted for by marked decreases in the HDL_{2b} subfraction.

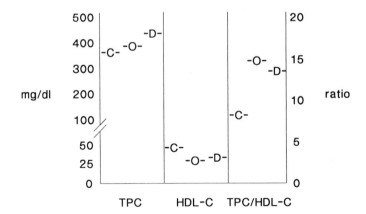

Figure 4. Treatment effects on plasma lipids for control (C), Ovral-treated (O) and Demulen-treated (D) cynomolgus females. Modified from Clarkson et al (1990).

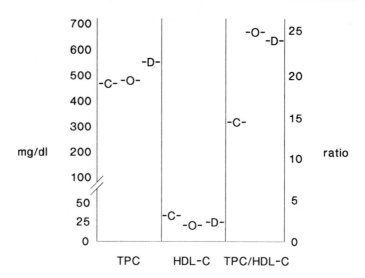

Figure 5. Treatment effects on plasma lipids for high risk (TPC/HDL-C>4.5) control (C), Ovral-treated (O) and Demulen-treated (D) cynomolgus females. Modified from Clarkson et al (1990).

Despite the marked lowering of HDL-C and the HDL_{2b} subfraction, and marked increases in TPC/HDL-C, the extent of coronary artery atherosclerosis was lessened by both contraceptive steroids, especially among females at high risk based on their plasma lipid profiles. The effect of these contraceptive steroids on coronary artery atherosclerosis extent are summarized in Figure 6.

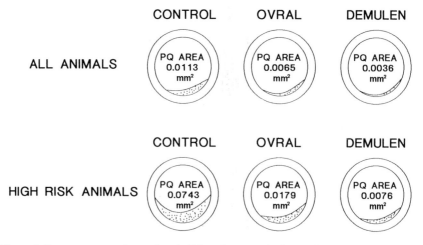

Figure 6. Coronary artery atherosclerosis (PQ = plaque area) of control animals, Ovral-treated and Demulen-treated cynomolgus females, both high risk animals (based on TPC/HDL-C) and all animals together. Modified from Clarkson et al (1990).

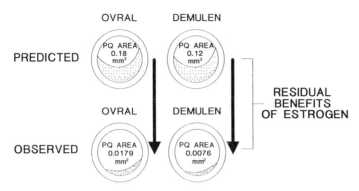

Figure 7. Schematic representation of the predicted coronary atherosclerosis outcomes based on plasma lipid/lipoprotein changes and the observed outcomes in the Demulen-treated and Ovral-treated animals. PQ = plaque area. Modified from Clarkson et al (1990).

A fascinating aspect of contraceptive steroid effects on coronary atherogenesis has been the disassociation between predicted (based on plasma lipids) and observed coronary artery plaque extent (Clarkson et al, 1990). In Figure 7 we have illustrated this disassociation.

Residual benefits of ethinyl oestradiol

The finding of a large inhibitory influence of the oral contraceptive treatments on initiation and progression of atherosclerosis was unexpected. In a previous study, treatment with an oral contraceptive preparation (Ovral) resulted in decreased coronary artery atherosclerosis when adjustment was made for plasma lipid changes. In that experiment, however, we did not attempt to estimate the 'residual effects' of the contraceptive preparation. Although we can estimate the size of the residual effect in this experiment (Figure 7), we cannot explain its mechanism(s). Clearly, steroid-induced changes in plasma lipid levels are not the same as changes induced by diet in terms of the promotion of atherogenesis. Furthermore, females at high risk for atherosclerosis due to their plasma lipid concentrations actually benefited the most from oral contraceptive treatment in terms of atherosclerosis extent, indicating that this effect is more than just a change in the relationship between plasma lipids and atherosclerosis. It seems likely that these beneficial residual effects are due to the ethinyl oestradiol component of the contraceptive steroids. There is considerable evidence to suggest that oestrogen affects atherogenesis independent of its effects on plasma lipid and lipoprotein concentrations. There is good evidence for the presence of oestrogen and progesterone receptors in arterial endothelium and smooth muscle cells in several mammalian species. Oestrogen treatment, based on both in vivo and in vitro studies, is associated with reductions in arterial smooth muscle cell proliferation, decreased collagen and elastin production, and increased degradation of collagen and elastin in arterial tissue.

There is additional indirect evidence for the beneficial effects of oestrogens on atherogenesis independent of plasma lipid and lipoprotein concentrations. In a previous study of contraceptive steroid effects on lipids and coronary artery atherosclerosis (Adams et al, 1987b), we compared the coronary atherosclerosis extent of a subset of control and oral contraceptive-treated female cynomolgus monkeys for which the ratio of TPC to HDL-C was less than 25. Females in the oral contraceptive group had less than one-fifth of the coronary artery atherosclerosis observed in the plasma lipid-matched control group. Interestingly, Bush and her colleagues (1987), studying cardiovascular disease incidence among women using oestrogen for reasons other than contraception, found indirect evidence of a protective effect of oestrogen after controlling for plasma lipid concentrations. Their results suggested that part of the beneficial effect of oestrogen use could be explained by changes in the plasma lipoproteins, but part of the benefit remained unexplained. Perhaps that unexplained portion is similar to what we have determined here as the residual effect of the contraceptive steroids, which we hypothesize is due to the ethinyl oestradiol component.

In seeking to determine the mechanism(s) that could account for this protective effect of ethinyl oestradiol, we used LDL labelled with tyramine cellobiose, a residualizing label, to measure the intracellular degradation and accumulation of LDL in arteries (Carew et al, 1984) of premenopausal cynomolgus females fed a moderately atherogenic diet for 16 weeks. Some of the observations from one of these studies are summarized in Figure 8.

Ovral and Triphasil induced a more 'atherogenic' lipid profile than diet alone, yet the accumulation of degradative products of LDL in the coronary arteries was significantly less (Figure 8) (J. D. Wagner et al, unpublished data).

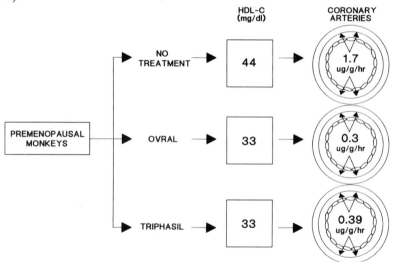

Figure 8. Mean HDL-C concentrations and coronary artery LDL accumulation in premenopausal cynomolgus females either not treated, treated with Ovral or treated with Triphasil. Modified from J. D. Wagner et al, unpublished data).

CHARACTERISTICS OF THE SURGICALLY POSTMENOPAUSAL CYNOMOLGUS FEMALE

Plasma lipid/lipoprotein changes and progression of coronary artery atherosclerosis

To understand better the social status-ovarian function interrelationships, we examined the influences of ovariectomy and social status on the extent of atherosclerosis in the cynomolgus macaque (Adams et al, 1985). Ovariectomy resulted in a more atherogenic plasma lipid pattern and much more extensive coronary artery atherosclerosis (Figure 9). Approximately one-half of the effect on atherosclerosis could be accounted for by effects on plasma lipids, with one-half remaining unexplained.

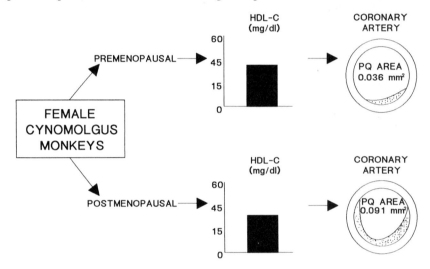

Figure 9. Plasma HDL-C concentrations and coronary artery atherosclerosis in premenopausal and surgically postmenopausal cynomolgus monkeys. PQ = plaque area. Modified from Adams et al (1985).

Increased bone turnover and loss of bone density/mineral

We have a decade or more of experience using cynomolgus macaques (*Macaca fascicularis*) as models for human atherosclerosis. More recently we have developed the surgically postmenopausal female cynomolgus macaque as a dual animal model useful for studying atherosclerosis and osteoporosis concurrently.

To study the effect of surgical menopause on bone mass, serial dual-photon absorptiometry (DPA) scans were done on female macaques that were subjects in a trial designed to examine the effect of oestrogen on established atherosclerosis (Jayo et al, 1990a). The lumbar vertebrae (L2–L4) were scanned in vivo premenopausally, and 1 year and 1½ years after surgical menopause. Lumbar spine bone mineral content and bone

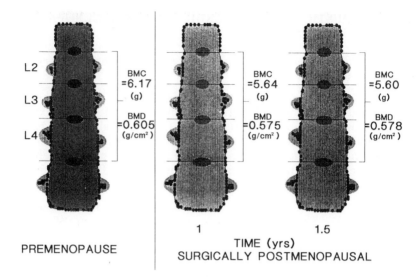

Figure 10. Bone mineral density (BMD) and bone mineral content (BMC) in lumbar vertebrae (L2–L4) of pre- and postmenopausal monkeys. BMD and BMC are decreased ($P < 0.001$). Data are adjusted means (covariates were body weight and the raw beam ratio of the dual-photon absorptiometry) (Jayo et al, 1990a).

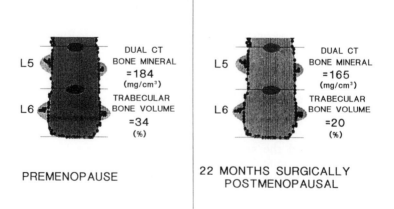

Figure 11. Bone mineral amount, as assessed by dual computed tomography (CT), of the fifth lumbar vertebra (L5) and trabecular bone volume (percent) of the sixth lumbar vertebra (L6) in premenopausal and surgically postmenopausal female macaques 22 months after ovariectomy. Modified from Miller et al (1986) and Mazess et al (1987).

mineral density decreased significantly with time (Jayo et al, 1990a) (Figure 10). These results suggest that surgically postmenopausal cynomolgus macaques mimic postmenopausal human primates in the loss of bone mass.

In an earlier study, we found that 22 months after induction of surgical menopause cynomolgus macaques had a lower vertebral radiographic density (Bowles et al, 1985), lower bone mineral content measured by computed tomography (Mazess et al, 1987) and lower trabecular bone volume (Miller et al, 1986) than premenopausal monkeys (Figure 11).

More recently, we scanned the entire thirteenth thoracic vertebra of these animals ex vivo using DPA (Model 2600, Norland, Inc., Fort Atkinson, Wisconsin) and dual-energy X-ray absorptiometry (DXA) (Model XR-26, Norland, Inc., Fort Atkinson, Wisconsin). Each bone was scanned using the spine scan mode with the bone placed on a water bath on a plexiglas sheet (Jayo et al, 1990b,c). Both methodologies detected significant decreases ($P < 0.05$) in bone mineral content and bone mineral density (with or without body weight as a covariate) in surgically postmenopausal compared with premenopausal female macaques.

Effects of surgical menopause on bone serum biomarkers

In a recent study, we compared the serum biomarkers of bone turnover (Welles et al, 1990) and in vivo and ex vivo bone densitometric values (Jayo et al, 1989) of premenopausal monkeys and monkeys surgically postmenopausal for 18 months. The groups were not significantly different ($P > 0.05$) in body weight, trunk length or body mass index. The serum biomarkers of bone turnover measured included total alkaline phosphatase, bone-specific alkaline phosphatase, acid phosphatase, tartrate-resistant acid phosphatase and osteocalcin (bone gla-protein).

Surgically postmenopausal monkeys had significantly lower ($P < 0.05$) lumbar spine bone mineral content and bone mineral density than premenopausal monkeys, as assessed by in vivo DPA.

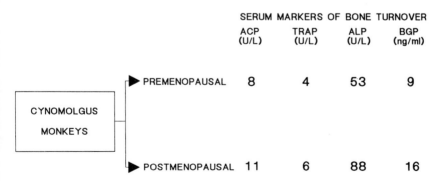

Figure 12. Serum biomarkers of bone turnover activity in postmenopausal monkeys (ACP = acid phosphatase; TRAP = tartrate-resistant acid phosphatase; ALP = alkaline phosphatase; BGP = bone gla-protein or osteocalcin). All are elevated ($P < 0.05$). Modified from Welles et al (1990).

Postmenopausal monkeys had significantly greater ($P<0.05$) levels of alkaline phosphatase, acid phosphatase, tartrate-resistant acid phosphatase and bone gla-protein than premenopausal macaques (Figure 12). All of the bone-related serum biomarkers indicated significantly greater bone turnover in postmenopausal monkeys compared with premenopausal monkeys.

OESTROGEN REPLACEMENT THERAPY AND THE POSTMENOPAUSAL CYNOMOLGUS FEMALE

Effect of parenteral oestradiol and progesterone on coronary artery atherosclerosis in surgically postmenopausal cynomolgus monkeys

We have reported the effects of physiological replacement of oestrogen (17β-oestradiol) alone and in combination with progesterone on coronary artery atherogenesis in surgically postmenopausal monkeys (hormones were administered subcutaneously in Silastic implants) (Adams et al, 1990). Physiological oestradiol replacement inhibited coronary artery atherosclerosis progression. The addition of progesterone did not diminish the beneficial effect of the oestradiol. The results are summarized in Figure 13.

In this study, the parenterally administered oestradiol had minimal effects on plasma lipoproteins. The oestradiol-induced lipoprotein changes accounted for only about 30% of the beneficial effect on coronary artery atherosclerosis (Figure 14). This observation is consistent with the findings of Bush and Miller-Bass (1990). The results of that meta-analysis, and our

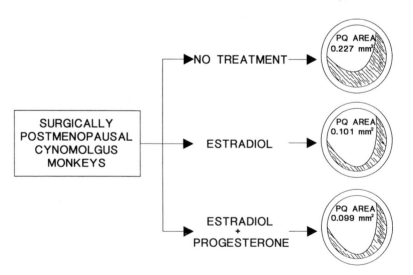

Figure 13. Coronary artery atherosclerosis extent in surgically postmenopausal monkeys receiving no hormone treatment, treatment with 17β-oestradiol or 17β-oestradiol plus progesterone. PQ = plaque area. Modified from Adams et al (1990).

study of monkeys, suggest that the beneficial effects of oestrogen on coronary atherosclerosis remain substantially unexplained by plasma lipoprotein changes (Figure 14).

We have used the trapped ligand, tyramine cellobiose, and methodology developed by Carew and colleagues (1984) to separately quantify LDL degradation and accumulation in coronary arteries. We studied coronary arteries of surgically postmenopausal cynomolgus monkeys fed an atherogenic diet and either treated or not treated with parenterally administered

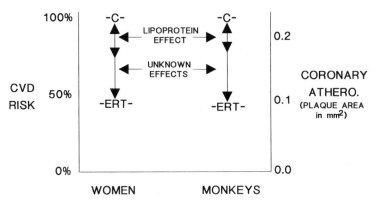

Figure 14. The extent to which the beneficial effects of oestrogen replacement on CVD in women and coronary artery atherosclerosis in cynomolgus monkeys can be explained by plasma lipoprotein changes and by other unknown effects. C = control (untreated); ERT = oestrogen replacement therapy. Modified from Adams et al (1990) and Bush and Miller-Bass (1990).

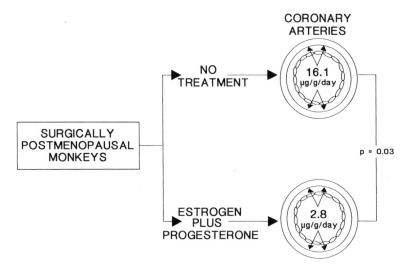

Figure 15. The effect of parenteral oestradiol (oestrogen) and progesterone replacement on the accumulation of LDL degradation products in the coronary arteries of surgically postmenopausal monkeys. Modified from Wagner et al (1989).

17 β-oestradiol and progesterone (Wagner et al, 1989). The findings are summarized in Figure 15.

The accumulation of LDL degradation products was greatly diminished by oestrogen replacement therapy. This finding indicates a mechanism by which oestrogen may inhibit atherogenesis directly at the level of the arterial intima, and account for unexplained variability in the effects of oestrogens and progestin on atherosclerosis and coronary heart disease risk.

Effect of parenteral oestradiol on endothelium-dependent vascular responses

Variant angina, due to coronary artery spasm, is believed to be more frequent in women than men. Because women, in general, have smaller coronary arteries related to their smaller body size, fluctuations in coronary tone may be of increased clinical importance. Atherosclerotic coronary arteries are susceptible to spasm induced by a wide variety of physiological stimuli such as exposure to cold, exercise and mental stress (Gage et al, 1986; Nabel et al, 1988; Rozanski et al, 1988). Additionally, atherosclerotic arteries are susceptible to spasm induced by endothelium-dependent vasoactive agents such as ergometrine (ergonovine *USP*), acetylcholine and products released by aggregating platelets and activated white blood cells (Henry and Yokoyama, 1980; Ludmer et al, 1986; Faraci et al, 1989; Lopez et al, 1989).

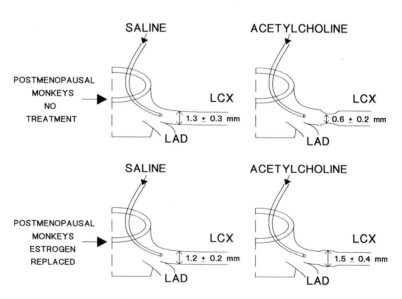

Figure 16. Coronary artery diameter response to intracoronary normal saline or acetylcholine in atherosclerotic, surgically postmenopausal monkeys, with or without oestrogen replacement therapy. LAD = left anterior descending coronary artery; LCX = left circumflex coronary artery. Modified from Williams et al (1990).

Oestrogen replacement may protect against coronary heart disease in menopausal women in two ways: (a) inhibition of coronary artery athero-sclerosis; and (b) preservation of normal expression of vascular responsiveness so that coronary blood flow is not inappropriately restricted by either attenuated dilator responses or augmented constrictor responses. Although the first mode of protection is recognized, at least experimentally, the effects of ovarian hormones on the dilator and constrictor responses of coronary arteries are less clear.

Using quantitative coronary angiography, we have examined the dilator responses of atherosclerotic coronary arteries to the intracoronary infusion of nitroglycerin and acetylcholine in surgically postmenopausal monkeys treated or not treated with parenteral oestradiol (Williams et al, 1990). Oestrogen administration did not change dilator responses to nitroglycerin but prevented paradoxical constriction to acetylcholine (Figure 16). Results indicate that oestrogen replacement protects against impaired endothelium-dependent dilatation in atherosclerotic coronary arteries, suggesting a potential role for oestrogen in the prevention of coronary artery spasm among oestrogen-deficient females.

Effects on bone of surgical menopause with or without hormonal therapy

The effects of oestrogen replacement therapy with or without progesterone on the skeletal and cardiovascular systems was evaluated 30 months after surgical menopause in macaques fed an atherogenic diet (Jayo et al, 1990c). We compared the ex vivo bone lumbar densitometric and histo-morphometric values of three groups of surgically postmenopausal monkeys: (a) untreated, (b) treated with oestrogen (17β-oestradiol) and progesterone, and (c) treated only with oestrogen (17β-oestradiol). Frozen serum samples, obtained at the time of necropsy, were analysed to determine serum biomarkers of bone turnover activity.

When covaried for body mass index, the bone mineral density of the third lumbar vertebral body, measured by DPA, was significantly lower in the untreated control group compared with the treated groups ($P = 0.018$). Bone mineral content was not significantly different between the groups, but the adjusted mean was greatest in the oestrogen plus progesterone group, followed closely by the oestrogen-treated group, and was least in the untreated group (Figure 17).

When covaried for body mass index, the trabecular bone volume of a midsagittal section of the first lumbar vertebra was not significantly different between the groups, but the adjusted mean was greatest in the oestrogen plus progesterone group, followed closely by the oestrogen-treated group, and was least in the untreated group. When covaried for body mass index, the trabecular plate number was significantly lower ($P = 0.022$) and the mean trabecular plate separation was significantly higher ($P = 0.033$) in the untreated group (Figure 17). Thus, both oestrogen and oestrogen plus progesterone provided overall protection against loss of bone postmeno-pausally.

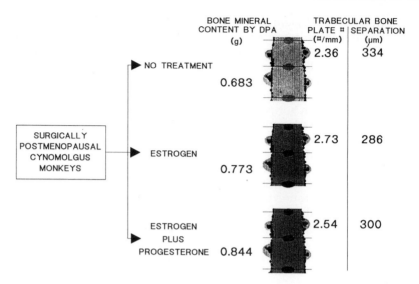

Figure 17. Bone mineral content, trabecular bone plate number and trabecular bone plate separation in surgically postmenopausal monkeys which were untreated, treated with oestrogen (17β-oestradiol) alone or with oestrogen plus progesterone. Modified from Jayo et al (1990c).

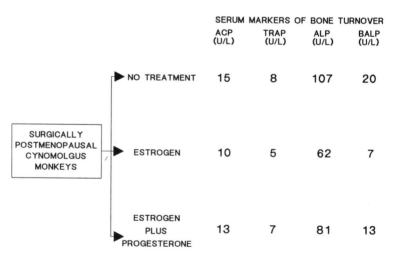

Figure 18. Serum biomarkers of bone turnover activity in surgically postmenopausal monkeys with and without hormone replacement (ACP = acid phosphatase; TRAP = tartrate-resistant acid phosphatase; ALP = alkaline phosphatase; BALP = bone ALP by wheat germ lectin binding). Modified from Welles et al (1990).

As expected, the ovariectomized animals had significant ($P < 0.05$) elevations of serum markers of bone turnover (Figure 18). These data demonstrate the clinical and histopathological similarity of the surgically postmenopausal cynomolgus macaque model of osteopenia and the osteoporosis of postmenopausal women.

SUMMARY

We have used the cynomolgus macaque as a model for the study of the effects of endogenous and exogenous sex steroid hormones on atherosclerosis and osteoporosis. As in human beings, premenopausal female cynomolgus macaques develop much less extensive coronary artery atherosclerosis than their male counterparts. Furthermore, surgical menopause results in a more atherogenic plasma lipoprotein pattern and an approximate doubling of atherosclerosis extent. Frequent pregnancy, a hyperoestrogenic state, results in an approximate 50% reduction in atherosclerosis extent. Physiological replacement with 17β-oestradiol alone or in combination with progesterone prevents the increase in coronary artery atherosclerosis extent associated with ovariectomy. This effect is independent of plasma lipoprotein concentrations and appears to be accounted for, at least in part, by an inhibitory effect of oestrogen replacement therapy on the uptake and degradation of LDL by the artery wall. Also, as in human beings, treatment with certain types of combination oral contraceptives results in marked decreases in plasma HDL-C concentration. Nonetheless, coronary artery atherosclerosis extent is reduced in monkeys by oral contraceptive treatment, and this effect is most pronounced among animals at highest risk due to theoretically adverse plasma lipoprotein profiles. It appears that, as with oestrogen replacement therapy, this effect can be accounted for, at least in part, by an inhibition of the uptake and degradation of low density lipoprotein by the artery wall.

The monkey also appears to be a good model for studies of postmenopausal bone loss. As in women, surgical menopause results in significant diminution of bone mineral density and bone mineral content. Also, serum biomarkers of bone turnover (total alkaline phosphatase, acid phosphatase, tartrate-resistant acid phosphatase and osteocalcin) are increased in surgically postmenopausal monkeys, indicating increased bone turnover resulting from the surgical menopause. These increases in bone loss and indices of bone turnover were prevented by physiological oestrogen replacement therapy.

Cynomolgus monkeys seem to be exceptionally useful models for studies of the effects of sex steroid hormones on atherosclerosis and osteoporosis, two major public health problems in postmenopausal women.

Acknowledgements

This work was supported by National Institutes of Health, National Heart, Lung, and Blood Institute Grants No. HL14164, HL33492 and HL38964, and Grant No. RR00919 of the

National Center for Research Resources of the National Institutes of Health. The authors gratefully acknowledge Martha Henderson for the clerical preparation of the manuscript and Ginger Petrick for her technical expertise in the preparation of the figures accompanying the manuscript.

REFERENCES

Adams MR, Rudel LL, Clarkson TB et al (1983) Influence of a levonorgestrel-containing contraceptive vaginal ring on plasma lipids and lipoproteins in cynomolgus monkeys. *Contraception* **28**: 253–266.

Adams MR, Kaplan JR, Clarkson TB & Koritnik DR (1985) Ovariectomy, social status, and atherosclerosis in cynomolgus monkeys. *Arteriosclerosis* **5**: 192–200.

Adams MR, Kaplan JR, Koritnik DR & Clarkson TB (1987a) Pregnancy-associated inhibition of coronary artery atherosclerosis in monkeys. Evidence of a relationship with endogenous estrogen. *Arteriosclerosis* **7**: 378–384.

Adams MR, Clarkson TB, Koritnik DR & Nash HA (1987b) Contraceptive steroids and coronary artery atherosclerosis of cynomolgus macaques. *Fertility and Sterility* **47**: 1010–1018

Adams MR, Kaplan JR, Manuck SB et al (1990) Inhibition of coronary artery atherosclerosis by 17-beta estradiol in ovariectomized monkeys: Lack of an effect of added progesterone. *Arteriosclerosis* **10**: 1051–1057.

Bowles EA, Weaver DS, Telewski FW et al (1985) Bone measurement by enhanced contrast image analysis: Ovariectomized and intact *Macaca fascicularis* as a model for human osteoporosis. *American Journal of Physiology and Anthropology* **67**: 99–103.

Bowman LA, Dilley SR & Keverne EB (1978) Suppression of oestrogen-induced LH surges by social subordination in talapoin monkeys. *Nature* **275**: 56–58.

Bush TL & Miller-Bass K (1990) Effect of hormone replacement on cardiovascular disease: an epidemiologic overview. In Christiansen C & Overgaard K (eds) *Osteoporosis 1990, Proceedings of the Third International Symposium on Osteoporosis*, pp 1817–1821. Copenhagen: Osteopress ApS.

Bush TL, Barrett-Connor E, Cowan LD et al (1987) Cardiovascular mortality and noncontraceptive use of estrogen in women: Results from the Lipid Research Clinics Program follow-up study. *Circulation* **75**: 1102–1109.

Carew TE, Pittman PC, Marchand ER & Steinberg D (1984) Measurement in vivo of irreversible degradation of low density lipoprotein in the rabbit aorta. Predominance of intimal degradation. *Arteriosclerosis* **4**: 214–224.

Christian JJ (1980) Endocrine factors in population regulation. In Cohen NN, Malpass RS & Klein HG (eds) *Biosocial Mechanisms of Population Regulation*, pp 55–116. New Haven: Yale University Press.

Clarkson TB, Hamm TE, Bullock BC & Lehner NDM (1976) Atherosclerosis in Old World monkeys. *Primates Medicine* **9**: 66–89.

Clarkson TB, Shively CA, Morgan TM et al (1990) Oral contraceptives and coronary artery atherosclerosis of cynomolgus monkeys. *Obstetrics and Gynecology* **75**: 217–222.

Dittus WPJ (1979) The evolution of behaviors regulating density and age-specific sex ratios in a primate population. *Behaviour* **69**: 265–302.

Drickamer LC (1974) A ten-year summary of reproductive data for free-ranging *Macaca mulatta*. *Folia Primatologica (Basel)* **21**: 61–80.

Faraci FM, Williams JK, Breese KR et al (1989) Atherosclerosis potentiates constrictor responses of cerebral and ocular blood vessels to thromboxane in monkeys. *Stroke* **20**: 242.

Gage E, Hess OM, Murakami J et al (1986) Vasoconstriction of stenotic coronary arteries during dynamic exercise in patients with classical angina pectoris; reversibility by nitroglycerin. *Circulation* **73**: 865–876.

Hamm TE Jr, Kaplan JR, Clarkson TB & Bullock BC (1983) Effects of gender and social behavior on the development of coronary artery atherosclerosis in cynomolgus macaques. *Atherosclerosis* **48**: 221–233.

Henry PO & Yokoyama M (1980) Supersensitivity of atherosclerotic rabbit aorta to ergonovine. *Journal of Clinical Investigation* **66**: 306–313.

Jayo MJ, Weaver DS, Adams MR & Rankin SE (1989) Anthropometry and bone mineral status in endocrinologically manipulated female cynomolgus macaques (*Macaca fascicularis*). *Journal of Bone and Mineral Research* 4: S181(abstract no. 256).

Jayo MJ, Weaver DS, Clarkson TB et al (1990a) Surgical menopause causes a significant decrease in lumbar bone mineral and serum HDL-cholesterol in female cynomolgus macaques. *Journal of Bone and Mineral Research* 5: S181(abstract no. 431).

Jayo MJ, Weaver DS, Rankin SE & Kaplan JR (1990b) Accuracy and reproducibility of lumbar bone mineral status determined by dual photon absorptiometry in live male cynomolgus macaques (*Macaca fascicularis*). *Laboratory Animal Science* 40(3): 266–269.

Jayo MJ, Weaver DS, Adams MR & Rankin SE (1990c) Effects on bone of surgical menopause and estrogen therapy with or without progesterone replacement in cynomolgus monkeys. *American Journal of Obstetrics and Gynecology* 163: 614–618.

Jewett DA & Dukelow WR (1972) Cyclicity and gestation length of *Macaca fascicularis*. *Primates* 13: 327–330.

Kannel WB, Castelli WP & Gordon T (1979) Cholesterol in the prediction of atherosclerotic disease. New perspectives based on the Framingham Study. *Annals of Internal Medicine* 90: 85–91.

Kaplan JR, Adams MR, Clarkson TB & Koritnik DR (1984) Psychosocial influences on female 'protection' among cynomolgus macaques. *Atherosclerosis* 53: 283–295.

Kaplan JR, Manuck SB, Clarkson TB & Prichard RW (1985) Animal models of behavioral influences on atherogenesis. *Advances in Behavioral Medicine* 1: 115–163.

Koritnik DR, Clarkson TB & Adams MR (1986) Cynomolgus macaques as models for evaluating effects of contraceptive steroids on plasma lipoproteins and coronary artery atherosclerosis. In Gregoire AT & Blye RP (eds) *Contraceptive Steroids: Pharmacology and Safety*, pp 303–319. New York: Plenum.

Lopez JAG, Armstrong ML, Harrison DG et al (1989) Vascular responses to leukocyte products in atherosclerotic primates. *Circulation Research* 65: 1078–1086.

Ludmer PL, Selwyn AP, Shook TL et al (1986) Paradoxical vasoconstriction induced by acetylcholine in atherosclerotic coronary arteries. *New England Journal of Medicine* 315: 1046–1051.

MacDonald GT (1971) Reproductive patterns of three species of macaques. *Fertility and Sterility* 22: 373–377.

Mahoney CJ (1970) A study of the menstrual cycle in *Macaca irus* with special reference to the detection of ovulation. *Journal of Reproduction and Fertility* 21: 153–163.

Mazess RB, Vetter J & Weaver DS (1987) Bone changes in oophorectomized monkeys: CT findings. *Journal of Computer Assisted Tomography* 11: 302–305.

Miller LC, Weaver DS, McAlister JA & Koritnik DR (1986) Effects of ovariectomy on vertebral trabecular bone in the cynomolgus monkey (*Macaca fascicularis*). *Calcified Tissue International* 38: 62–65.

Nabel EG, Ganz P, Gordon JB et al (1988) Dilation of normal and constriction of atherosclerotic coronary arteries caused by the cold pressor test. *Circulation* 77: 43–52.

Parks JS, Pelkey SJ, Babiak J & Clarkson TB (1989) Contraceptive steroid effects on lipids and lipoproteins in cynomolgus monkeys. *Arteriosclerosis* 9: 261–268.

Rozanski A, Bairy CN, Krantz DS et al (1988) Mental stress and the induction of silent myocardial ischemia in patients with coronary artery diease. *New England Journal of Medicine* 318: 1005–1012.

Sade DS, Cushing K, Cushing P et al (1976) Population dynamics in relation to social structure on Cayo Santiago. *Yearbook of Physiology and Anthropology* 20: 253–262.

Silk JB, Clark-Wheatley CB, Rodman PS & Samuels A (1981) Differential reproductive success and facultative adjustment of sex ratios among captive female bonnet macaques (*Macaca radiata*). *Animal Behaviour* 29: 1106–1120.

Tejada C, Strong JP, Montenegro MR, Restrepo C & Solberg LA (1968) Distribution of coronary and aortic atherosclerosis by geographic location, race, and sex. *Laboratory Investigation* 18: 509–526.

Tikkanen MJ & Nikkila EA (1986) Oral contraceptives and lipoprotein metabolism. *Journal of Reproductive Medicine* 31: 898–905.

Wagner JD, Clarkson TB, St Clair RW et al (1991) Estrogen and progesterone replacement therapy reduces low density lipoprotein accumulation in the coronary arteries of surgically postmenopausal cynomolgus monkeys. *Journal of Clinical Investigation* 84 (in press).

Walker ML, Gordon TP & Wilson ME (1983) Menstrual cycle characteristics of seasonally breeding rhesus monkeys. *Biology of Reproduction* **29:** 841–848.

Welles EG, Jayo MJ, Weaver DS, Carlson CS & Rankin SE (1990) Characterization of serum chemistry markers of bone turnover in surgically postmenopausal cynomolgus macaques. *Journal of Bone and Mineral Research* **5:** S182(abstract no. 432).

Williams JK, Adams MR & Klopfenstein HS (1990) Estrogen modulates responses of atherosclerotic coronary arteries. *Circulation* **81(5):** 1680–1687.

Wilson ME, Gordon TP & Bernstein IS (1978) Timing of births and reproductive success in rhesus monkey social groups. *Journal of Medical Primatology* **7:** 202–212.

11

Prevention of osteoporotic fractures: what we need to know

S. R. CUMMINGS

LIMITATIONS OF THE CLINICAL MODEL

Clinical research in osteoporosis is oriented to the care of individual patients with osteoporosis. From this perspective, the most effective approach to the prevention of fractures is to investigate potential aetiologies for osteoporosis, treat underlying causes and prescribe the most effective available therapies. This leads to research that focuses on the pathophysiology of osteoporosis and the development of potent treatments for bone loss. The primary goals are generally to maintain or increase bone mass in an individual. The effectiveness of treatment is the paramount concern.

Fractures are also a public health problem. In some regions of the world, as many as half of all women will suffer a fracture at some time in life and about one in six will suffer a hip fracture (Cummings et al, 1989). Even in countries with sophisticated medical systems, accepted clinically based programmes for evaluation and treatment often reach only a minority of those who might benefit. The potential costs of universal clinical evaluation and long-term pharmacological treatment to prevent fractures are prohibitive. Thus, we cannot rely on the classical clinical model to substantially reduce the incidence of fractures.

Viewing osteoporosis as a public health problem is necessary in trying to substantially reduce the incidence of fractures. From this perspective, people who do not visit a physician are as important as those who do, and the effectiveness of treatment is only one consideration. Questions of equal importance include: How common are risk factors that can be effectively changed? How many people can be reached with an intervention? How much disability, death and cost can be prevented in the population in return for the costs?

During the next decade, we may have enough information to design programmes capable of preventing a substantial proportion of fractures. For this to happen it will be necessary to have a systematic approach. This chapter proposes such an approach and points out the type of information that is needed to devise effective programmes for preventing fractures in populations.

AN APPROACH TO ASSESSING THE IMPACT OF INTERVENTIONS

How much suffering, disability, death and cost can be prevented by a programme to prevent fractures? How many fractures will be prevented? The answer can be estimated from several types of data. The reduction in the incidence of a fracture that could result from an intervention to change a risk factor (such as low dietary calcium intake) is a product of five factors: (a) the incidence of the fracture in those without that risk factor (I); (b) the prevalence of the risk factor (P); (c) the relative risk of fracture due to that condition (RR); (d) the proportional reduction in the incidence of the fracture due to an intervention (k), and (e) the applicability of the treatment (A), for example, the proportion of people with low calcium intake who are reached by the programme and who increase their calcium intake sufficiently to reduce their risk of fracture. Browner (1986) has put this in mathematical terms:

$$\text{Preventable risk} = I \times P \times RR \times k \times A \qquad \text{(Equation 1)}$$

Since the reduction in the incidence of fractures is the product of these factors, all are equally important. Doubling any one of the factors will double the impact of the programme.

The goal of prevention of fractures is to prevent pain, disability, death and economic costs. These consequences differ according to the type of fracture. On average, prevention of hip fractures, for example, will prevent more disability, death and medical cost than prevention of other types of fractures. Prevention of these consequences can be estimated by adding a sixth term to the equation—the average consequence (C, in terms of days of disability, years of life expectancy lost, or costs) attributable to the type of fracture:

$$\text{Preventable consequences} = I \times P \times RR \times k \times A \times C \qquad \text{(Equation 2)}$$

Many of these factors are known for hip fractures. The incidence of hip fractures has been described for most European countries and the United States. Several preventable risk factors for hip fractures have been found (Kelsey et al, 1990). Long-term use of oestrogen and, perhaps, thiazide diuretics reduce the risk of hip fracture by about 40–50% (Ray et al, 1989a). In contrast, there have been fewer good studies of other types of fractures and very few concerned with their consequences. There has been virtually no work on how to increase the applicability of interventions. This is unfortunate because doubling the applicability of an effective intervention will prevent as many fractures as finding a new treatment that is twice as effective in reducing the risk.

These equations serve as an outline for surveying what we know and what we need to find out in order to estimate the impact of programmes to prevent fractures.

INCIDENCE OF FRACTURES

The age-specific incidence of hip fractures is now known for most areas of the world that have universal access to hospitals, keep reliable records of hospitalization, and have an accurate census. The incidence is greatest in elderly Caucasian women in Northern Europe and North America. Within these areas there is regional variation (Melton, 1990). The incidence of hip fracture is highest in nursing homes (Lauritzen et al, 1990) and urban areas (Gärdsell et al, 1990). The incidence of hip fracture in Asia has now been studied (Orimo et al, 1990). It is lower in Japan than in North America and Northern Europe. Hip fractures appear to have become a much more important problem in Hong Kong; the incidence appears to have risen dramatically during the past 30 years and is now similar to that of Caucasians in Northern Europe and North America (Lau et al, 1990). No data is available for the People's Republic of China, Middle Eastern countries or Africa.

The incidence of vertebral fractures is difficult to assess because many occur asymptomatically and there is controversy about how to define them (Melton, 1987). Melton et al (1989) has suggested that the annual incidence of vertebral fractures among white women in the United States is about 2–3% per year after the age of 70, but the definitions of vertebral fracture used in that cross-sectional survey may have substantially overestimated the actual incidence (Smith-Bindman et al, 1991).

Most types of non-spine fractures are related to reduced bone mineral density (Seeley et al, 1990), but the incidence of these types of fractures has not been adequately studied even in the United States or Northern Europe.

PREVALENCE AND RELATIVE RISK OF MODIFIABLE RISK FACTORS

There have been a few prospective studies of common risk factors for fractures; most of these have focused on hip fractures. There have been very few prospective studies of risk factors for vertebral or other types of non-spine fractures (Kelsey et al, 1990).

The effect of changing a risk factor for fractures depends on both the strength of the risk factor (indicated by its relative risk) and its prevalence. Elimination of some well-established modifiable risk factors that affect a relatively small proportion of people would prevent only a small percentage of hip fractures. For example, use of long-acting sedative hypnotic or psychotropic drugs increases the risk of hip fractures by a factor of 1.7 (Ray et al, 1989b). Theoretically, if a woman stops using long-acting sedatives, she reduces her risk of hip fracture by 70%. But fewer than 5% of women use long-acting sedatives, so their complete elimination would reduce the incidence of hip fractures by less than 3.5%.

To develop more effective approaches to reducing the number of fractures, it is important to find common modifiable risk factors for hip, spine and other types of fractures. In particular, commonly used medications that might affect bone metabolism (such as non-steroidal anti-inflammatory drugs) and dietary constituents are important topics of study.

In addition, studies of risk factors for fractures that involve falls should focus on common modifiable risk factors for falls, such as footwear.

The strength and prevalence of risk factors are likely to vary from region to region. For example, dietary calcium deficiency is uncommon in Scandinavia and, thus, if calcium deficiency increases the risk of fracture, campaigns to increase calcium supplementation in Scandinavia will prevent few fractures. In contrast, the average intake of calcium in Hong Kong is very low (Lau et al, 1990), and programmes to increase calcium supplementation in that population are likely to prevent more fractures.

EFFICACY OF INTERVENTIONS

Long-term use of oestrogen therapy reduces the risk of hip, wrist and spine fractures by about 50% (Ray et al, 1989b). Etidronate appears to reduce the incidence of new vertebral deformities by about 50% (Storm et al, 1990); to estimate the potential impact of bisphosphonates or other treatments there is a need for controlled trials of their effectiveness for non-spine fractures.

There is little information about the effectiveness of interventions that could be applied to a large proportion of a population. Specifically, the effectiveness of increasing calcium intake and of simple but feasible exercise programmes, like daily walking, need to be studied. Intensive interventions that can be applied to patients in clinics can be tested in small randomized trials, but these tend to have insufficient statistical power for studying widely applicable interventions such as walking. To determine their effect on rates of fracture will require very large studies that will be feasible only if the interventions and assessments of outcomes are simple and inexpensive.

APPLICABILITY

Effective treatments will have little impact on the incidence of fractures if they reach only a small proportion of people at risk of fracture. For example, even though long-term oestrogen therapy reduces the risk of hip fracture by 50%, fewer than 15% of older women in the US are receiving oestrogen (Cauley et al, 1990). Thus current patterns of oestrogen use reduce the incidence of hip fracture in the US by less than 7.5%. The possibility that thiazide diuretics might prevent fractures is important because they are probably applicable to a larger proportion of women than oestrogen (about one-third of elderly women in the US already take thiazide diuretics) and to men. If thiazide diuretics reduce the risk of fracture by 40%, then current patterns of use of thiazides reduce the incidence of hip fracture in women by about 13%.

The effectiveness of interventions has received considerable study, but virtually no attention has been paid to methods of increasing the applicability of effective treatments. For example, about 50% of women given a prescription for oestrogen either do not fill it or stop taking it within a year; by reducing the applicability of treatment, these decisions to avoid or stop treatment reduce the potential impact of oestrogen by at least half. Nevertheless, there has been little study of the reasons why physicians do not offer hormone therapy and why women do not take hormone therapy, and there have been no trials of methods to increase physicians' prescription of and women's use of postmenopausal oestrogen.

Densitometry identifies women at risk of fracture, but it may also be a powerful tool for increasing the adoption of measures to prevent fractures. Rubin and Cummings (1990) found that women whose bone densitometry results were below normal were much more likely to start taking oestrogen, increase their calcium intake, start exercising regularly, and even take precautions to prevent falls. Results of densitometry might also reduce rates of fractures by improving compliance with long-term therapy. This potential effect of densitometry may be as important to study as its ability to predict fractures.

Non-compliance is one of the most important barriers to the application of preventive measures to large populations. Education and publicity have had important but limited impacts in other areas of prevention, such as the use of seat belts. Changes in the environment that do not require individual compliance (like requiring air bags in cars) could substantially increase the applicability and impact of an intervention. Thus, fortification of the water supply with calcium (Rodrigues et al, 1990) will generally have more impact than educational campaigns to encourage individuals to increase their calcium intake.

Environmental modifications may be especially promising for the prevention of hip fractures due to falls in nursing homes or group housing designed for the elderly, where these modifications can be applied universally. For example, Buchner has observed that falls on concrete, hardwood or tile surfaces (ubiquitous in US nursing homes) are about five times as likely to result in hip fractures as falls on softer surfaces (D. Buchner, personal communication). Universal installation of softer floor covering could prevent as many as 80% of hip fractures in those residences.

CONSEQUENCES OF FRACTURES

Estimating the effect of interventions on costs, disability or death due to osteoporosis requires better information about the consequences of all types of fractures. Two issues deserve study. First, hip fractures are commonly followed by severe consequences, but it is not known how much of the death, disability and costs of care are attributable to the fracture (and are thus preventable by avoiding the fracture) and how much is attributable to comorbid conditions that increase the risk of death, disability and hip fracture. Browner et al (1990) has observed that women with low bone mass have an increased mortality rate from causes besides fracture, suggesting that some osteoporotic fractures might be the manifestation of chronic illness or frailty. If so, treatment to slow bone loss alone may have less impact on function and survival than would be predicted from the prevention of fracture.

Second, very little is known about the consequences of other fractures that are associated with reduced bone mass. The pain, disability and costs attributable to vertebral fractures are uncertain and the consequences of non-spine fractures besides hip fractures have not been adequately studied (Cummings, 1987). This information is essential to estimating the potential benefits and cost-effectiveness of various programmes to prevent fractures.

AN EXAMPLE

To illustrate this approach, consider the impact of a programme to screen postmenopausal women with densitometry and treat the one-third ($P = 0.33$) with the lowest bone mineral density with oestrogen. Assume that 500 hip fractures occur each year in a population of 100 000 postmenopausal women ($I = 0.005$), similar to the rate found in the United States and Northern Europe. Assume that the women whose bone mass is in the lowest third have twice the lifetime risk of fracture ($RR = 2$) as other women (Black et al, 1990). Taken long-term, oestrogen reduces the risk of hip fractures by 50% ($k = 0.5$). The most uncertain factor is the applicability of this programme. Assume (optimistically) that 50% of women could be reached with screening and (optimistically) that 40% would take oestrogen long term. Overall, the applicability (A) of this programme would be $0.5 \times 0.4 = 0.2$. Using Equation 1:

Reduction in hip fracture incidence $= 0.005 \times 0.33 \times 2 \times 0.5 \times 0.2 = 0.00033$

This programme would (at best) eventually prevent only 33 of the 500 hip fractures per year in a population of 100 000 women. The impact could be enhanced by finding ways to increase its applicability by increasing the number of women screened and the proportion of women who comply with long-term treatment. Thus, these areas should have a high research priority.

Using this approach Browner (1990) has demonstrated how a high risk strategy for screening and treating one-third of women who have low bone mass with oestrogen may prevent a slightly smaller proportion of hip fractures (6%) than a population strategy of universally applied (but less effective) calcium supplementation (8%). This example illustrates that the impact of a strategy depends as much on the applicability of an intervention as on its effectiveness.

THE NON-SPECIFICITY PRINCIPLE

In designing interventions to prevent non-spine fractures it is commonly believed that the intervention should be specific to the reason for the increased risk. In this approach, a woman who has an increased risk of falling but normal bone mass should have a treatment that focuses on the prevention of falls, not on prevention of bone loss. In contrast, the approach outlined in this chapter implies that the treatment need not be specific to the cause of the increased risk; effectiveness, not means of action, is what counts. High risk individuals will benefit from the most effective interventions, regardless of the reason for their increased risk. Thus, for hip fractures, women who are most osteopenic have the most to gain from prevention of falls, even if they have a normal risk of falling. Conversely, women who are at greatest risk of falling may have the most to gain by treatments to slow bone loss, even if their bone mass is within the normal range. Assessments of bone mass and of risk of falls are complementary and efforts to prevent osteopenia and trauma are likely to have at least additive impacts for the prevention of fractures that result from both osteopenia and trauma.

DIRECTIONS FOR RESEARCH

To persuade policy-makers that efforts to prevent fractures are worthwhile there is a need for better data about the incidence and consequences of fractures besides fractures of the hip. In addition, the types of findings that are likely to have the greatest impact include:

1. Discovery of changes in the risk of fractures associated with very common exposures, such as widely used medications or ubiquitous environmental factors, such as concrete or tile flooring.
2. Demonstration of the efficacy of interventions that are feasible for widespread applicability, such as dietary supplementation, simple forms of exercise and energy-absorbing flooring or clothing. This will require large scale, simple randomized trials.
3. Development of ways to increase the adoption of and compliance with preventive measures, such as oestrogen therapy, that can effectively reduce the risk of fractures.

REFERENCES

Black DM, Melton LJ III & Cummings SR (1990) In Christiansen C & Overgaard K (eds) *Osteoporosis 1990*, p 861. Osteopress Aps.
Browner WS (1986) *American Journal of Epidemiology* **123:** 143.
Browner WS (1990) In Christiansen C & Overgaard K (eds) *Osteoporosis 1990*, p 1123. Osteopress Aps.
Browner WS, Seeley DC, Black D, Cauley J, Hulley SB & Cummings SR (1990) In Christiansen C & Overgaard K (eds) *Osteoporosis 1990*, p 71. Osteopress Aps.
Cauley J, Cummings SR, Black DM, Mascioli SR & Seeley DG (1990) *American Journal of Obstetrics and Gynecology* **163:** 1438.
Cummings SR (1987) In Christiansen C, Overgaard K, Johansen JS & Riis BNJ (eds) *Osteoporosis 1987*, p 1193. Osteopress Aps.
Cummings SR, Black D & Rubin SM (1989) *Archives of Internal Medicine* **149:** 2445.
Gärdsell P, Johnell O, Nilsson BE & Sernbo I (1990) In Overgaard K et al (eds) *Third International Symposium on Osteoporosis*, abstract 46.
Kelsey JL, Grisso JA & Maggi S (1990) In Christiansen C & Overgaard K (eds) *Osteoporosis 1990*, p 62. Osteopress Aps.
Lau EMC, Cooper C, Donnan S & Barker DJP. In Christiansen C & Overgaard K (eds) *Osteoporosis 1990*, p 66. Osteopress Aps.

Lauritzen JB, Petersen MM & Lund B. In Christiansen C & Overgaard K (eds) *Osteoporosis 1990*, p 152. Osteopress Aps.
Melton LJ (1987) In Christiansen C, Overgaard K, Johansen JS & Riis BNJ (eds) *Osteoporosis 1987,* p 33. Osteopress Aps.
Melton LJ III (1990) In Christiansen C & Overgaard K (eds) *Osteoporosis 1990*, p 36. Osteopress Aps.
Melton LJ, Kan SH, Frye MA, Wahner HW, O'Fallon WM & Riggs BL (1989) *American Journal of Epidemiology* **129:** 1000.
Orimo H, Hosoi T, Nakamura T, Ouchi Y & Shiraki M (1990) In Christiansen C & Overgaard K (eds) *Osteoporosis 1990*, p 55. Osteopress Aps.
Ray WA, Downey W, Griffin MR & Melton LJ (1989a) *Lancet* **i:** 687.
Ray WA, Griffin MR & Downey W (1989b) *Journal of the American Medical Association* **262:** 3303.
Rodrigues M, Branco JC, Menezes V, Neves LC, Fernandes JJ & Queiroz MV (1990) In Christiansen C & Overgaard K (eds) *Osteoporosis 1990*, p 175. Osteopress Aps.
Rubin SM & Cummings SR (1990) In Christiansen C & Overgaard K (eds) *Osteoporosis 1990*, p 1125. Osteopress Aps.
Seeley DG, Browner WS, Nevitt MC, Genant HK & Scott JC (1990) In Christiansen C & Overgaard K (eds) *Osteoporosis 1990*, p 463. Osteopress Aps.
Smith-Bindman R, Cummings SR, Steiger P & Genant HK (1991) *Journal of Bone and Mineral Research* **6:** 25.
Storm T, Thamsborg G, Steiniche T, Genant HK & Sørenson OH (1990) *New England Journal of Medicine* **322:** 1265.

12

Cost-effectiveness of hormone replacement
therapy after the menopause

ANNA N. A. TOSTESON
MILTON C. WEINSTEIN

Assessing the role of hormone replacement therapy in the menopause is a
complex undertaking. To evaluate the appropriate role for hormone
replacement therapy in a society of limited resources, individual patient's
net health benefits from therapy must be considered in relation to society's
net resource costs. Included in the benefits of therapy are the preservation of
bone density and the corresponding reduction in the risk of osteoporotic
fractures of the wrist, femur and vertebrae, as well as a potential reduction in
ischaemic heart disease incidence and death. Among the potential risks of
therapy are the development of endometrial and breast cancers. The
resource costs associated with each component of risk are great, as are the
costs of hormone replacement therapy. Based on United States census
projections, Weinstein and Tosteson (1990) estimate that the cost of treating
postmenopausal US women aged 50–64 years with hormone replacement
therapy alone would range from 3.5 to 5 billion dollars annually.

In this chapter, using the framework of cost-effectiveness analysis, data
from the clinical and epidemiological literature are combined with economic
data to assess both net health benefits and net direct medical costs for several
management strategies involving hormone replacement therapy. Analyses
by Weinstein and Tosteson (1990), Weinstein and Schiff (1982) and
Weinstein (1980) have evaluated the cost-effectiveness of prescribing
hormone replacement therapy for all women in the menopause. A recent
paper by Tosteson et al (1990) also evaluated the cost-effectiveness of
screening perimenopausal women on the basis of bone mineral density of
the femur to target hormone replacement therapy at women at highest risk
of hip fracture. Here we update and integrate data from these and other
sources to reflect current medical practice and current understanding of the
risks and benefits of hormone replacement therapy. For each management
strategy we ask: at what cost is the additional benefit achieved?

HORMONE REPLACEMENT THERAPY REGIMENS

We address the clinical management of perimenopausal women who have had a previous hysterectomy separately from perimenopausal women with an intact uterus. For both populations, a strategy of no intervention is the baseline from which comparisons with other strategies are made. For women with a previous hysterectomy, 10- and 15-year courses of unopposed oestrogen consisting of 0.625 mg/day of conjugated oestrogen are considered. For women with intact uteri, a progestin is added to the treatment regimen to counteract the increase in endometrial hyperplasia and cancer that is associated with unopposed oestrogen, as shown in a recent study by Persson et al (1989) and as reviewed by Ziel (1982). Thus, 10- and 15-year courses of combined oestrogen with progestin, consisting of 25 days of 0.625 mg/day of conjugated oestrogen followed by 10 days of 10 mg/day of progestin, are evaluated for women with intact uteri. Shorter treatment durations were not evaluated because an analysis by Tosteson et al (1990) indicated that shorter durations are cost-ineffective when prevention of osteoporosis is a primary objective. Although widespread use of hormone replacement therapy has not been advocated by the US Preventive Services Task Force (1990) or others, these treatment regimens reflect current clinical practice as documented in Utian's (1988) consensus statement on progestin use in postmenopausal women. Note that for the patient populations defined, none of the hormone replacement regimens require regular endometrial monitoring.

To fully evaluate the role of hormone replacement therapy in the light of currently available technology for measuring bone mineral density, we also discuss several screening strategies, which were evaluated by Tosteson et al (1990). These strategies allow for a single measurement of bone mineral density of the femur using dual-photon absorptiometry at age 50 years followed by 10 or 15 years of hormone replacement therapy in women who were determined to be 'at high risk' for hip fracture on the basis of their bone mineral measurement.

ENDPOINTS FOR COST-EFFECTIVENESS EVALUATION

Net health benefit

For each management strategy, net health benefit, or overall effectiveness, is measured from the patient's perspective and is represented either as the change in life expectancy (dLE) or the change in quality-adjusted life expectancy ($dQALE$). When life expectancy is used, the components of net health benefit represent changes in life expectancy due to changes in hip fracture incidence ($\pm dLE_{HFX}$), breast cancer incidence ($\pm dLE_{BRCA}$) and ischaemic heart disease death ($\pm dLE_{IHD}$). When quality-adjusted life expectancy is used, additional components represent changes in quality of life due to acute hip fracture incidence, disability and nursing home residency ($\pm dQ_{HFX}$), and symptom relief or discomfort resulting from hormone replacement therapy ($\pm dQ_{SYMPT}$).

Net resource cost

Net resource costs (dC) to society were estimated from direct medical costs or charges when cost data were unavailable. The components of cost include the costs of acute hip fracture ($\pm dC_{\text{HFX}}$), long-term nursing home stays ($\pm dC_{\text{NH}}$), breast cancer ($\pm dC_{\text{BRCA}}$) and hormone replacement therapy ($\pm dC_{\text{HRT}}$). All direct medical costs are considered regardless of the payer. Thus, the analysis reflects a societal perspective.

Cost-effectiveness ratios

The cost-effectiveness ratios (dC/dLE and $dC/dQALE$) are defined as:

$$\frac{dC}{dLE} = \frac{dC_{\text{HRT}} \pm dC_{\text{NH}} \pm dC_{\text{BRCA}} \pm dC_{\text{HFX}}}{\pm dLE_{\text{HFX}} \pm dLE_{\text{BRCA}} \pm dLE_{\text{IHD}}}$$

and

$$\frac{dC}{dQALE} = \frac{dC_{\text{HRT}} \pm dC_{\text{NH}} \pm dC_{\text{BRCA}} \pm dC_{\text{HFX}}}{\pm dLE_{\text{HFX}} \pm dLE_{\text{BRCA}} \pm dLE_{\text{IHD}} \pm dQ_{\text{HFX}} \pm dQ_{\text{SYMPT}}}$$

As described by Eisenberg (1989), incremental cost-effectiveness ratios represent the additional costs and benefits obtained for one strategy in comparison to the next most costly alternative strategy. These ratios provide a common metric with which policy analysts can evaluate and compare the relative value of health interventions. In this chapter, incremental cost-effectiveness ratios comparing hormone replacement therapy with no intervention are presented. In addition, when less costly screen-and-treat strategies are considered, the incremental ratios for hormone replacement therapy are computed relative to the next most costly screening strategy. All endpoints in the analysis are discounted at a rate of 5% per year. The effect of discounting, as described by Weinstein and Stason (1977), is to value future years of life and costs less heavily than those encountered in the near-term.

MARKOV STATE-TRANSITION MODEL

The utility of Markov state-transition models for following theoretical cohorts of patients over time to assess prognosis has been discussed by Beck and Pauker (1983). To assess the impact that hormone replacement therapy has on model endpoints through its impact on hip fracture incidence and sequelae, ischaemic heart disease deaths and quality of life we used the Markov state-transition model previously described by Tosteson et al (1990). The model, which assumes that all women are initially well and living in the community, followed women from age 50 to 100 years and kept an annual account of hip fracture incidence, placement in a nursing home, and deaths from hip fracture, ischaemic heart disease and other causes. Because breast cancer was not originally included in the model, a separate analysis estimated the excess mortality from breast cancer when hormone replacement therapy was modelled as a risk factor for breast cancer.

DATA AND ASSUMPTIONS

Hip fracture

Intertrochanteric and cervical hip fracture incidence was modelled as a function of bone mineral density and age according to a multiple regression model derived by Melton et al (1988) from a population-based survey of women in Rochester, Minnesota. Our model assumed that the initial distribution of bone mineral density by age followed that reported by Melton et al (1986) for women 45 to 54 years of age, where the average of the cervical and intertrochanteric bone density distributions was used. Without hormone replacement therapy, bone loss in the menopause was modelled as a quadratic function of age, which was described by Melton et al (1988) as follows:

$$\Delta BMD_{\text{cervical}} = (0.411171 \times 10^{-1}) - (0.169617 \times 10^{-2} \times \text{age}) + (0.135478 \times 10^{-4} \times \text{age}^2)$$

$$\Delta BMD_{\text{intertrochanteric}} = (0.368755 \times 10^{-1}) - (0.144192 \times 10^{-2} \times \text{age}) + (0.110406 \times 10^{-4} \times \text{age}^2)$$

Thus, as the cohort of 50-year-old women ages, the model calculates an updated bone mineral density for each individual, which determines her probability of hip fracture in the subsequent year.

Hormone replacement therapy has been shown by Quigley et al (1987), Ettinger et al (1985) and others to stop or slow bone loss in menopausal women. We assumed that women receiving hormone replacement therapy would sustain no loss in bone density. Based on reports by Christiansen et al (1981) and Lindsay et al (1978), following termination of therapy we assumed that bone loss resumed and continued at the same rate that it would have at menopause in the absence of hormone replacement therapy.

Using this model and assumptions, Tosteson et al (1990) reported a cumulative incidence of hip fracture of 17% in women who received no hormone replacement therapy and a cumulative incidence of 9% in women who received a 15-year course of oestrogen-progestin therapy. These projections are consistent with other population-based estimates, such as the 16% lifetime risk of hip fracture in untreated women that was estimated by Cummings et al (1989). Tosteson et al (1990) were also able to simulate the long-term oestrogen exposures seen in two epidemiological studies and to adequately reproduce the relative risks for hip fracture in treated versus untreated women that were reported by Weiss et al (1980) and Kiel et al (1987).

Sequelae of hip fracture

An increase in mortality following hip fracture has been shown by Pettiti and Sidney (1989), Weiss et al (1983) and others, and this excess mortality rises with age. An increase in mortality with increasing comorbidity has also been well established by Mossey et al (1989), Kenzora et al (1984), Kreutzfeld et al (1984), Dahl (1980) and Miller (1978). As described by Tosteson et al (1990), we assumed that 50% of the age-specific mortality observed in the year following hip fracture in the population from Rochester, Minnesota was attributable to the hip fracture.

Probabilities of entering a nursing home after a hip fracture were obtained from the 1984 National Hospital Discharge Survey, with adjustment to account for an estimated 34% of admissions that are discharged within 1 year. When computing quality-adjusted life expectancy, we assumed, as did Hillner et al (1986), that the probability of being disabled (i.e. free-living, but not in prefracture state of health) at 1 year after fracture was equal to the probability of remaining in a nursing home. Note that a distinction between the disabled and well health states is made only when quality of life is evaluated. The probabilities of attaining each health state at 1 year after a hip fracture are summarized in Table 1.

Table 1. Probability of being in each health state at 1 year after hip fracture.

Age group	Health state at 1 year following hip fracture*			
	Dead	NH†	Dis‡	Well§
50–59	0.06	0.0	0.0	0.94
60–64	0.03	0.14	0.14	0.69
65–69	0.03	0.19	0.19	0.59
70–74	0.06	0.24	0.24	0.46
75–79	0.06	0.25	0.25	0.44
80–84	0.11	0.31	0.31	0.27
85+	0.11	0.30	0.30	0.29

* The numbers in this table are rounded.
† Nursing home residency.
‡ Disabled and residing at home.
§ Returned to prefracture state.

Ischaemic heart disease

The importance of heart disease in evaluating the role of hormone replacement therapy in the menopause has been shown by Tosteson et al (1990), Henderson et al (1988) and Hillner et al (1986). The association between hormone replacement therapy and ischaemic heart disease in menopausal women has been the focus of many investigations. As reviewed by Bush (1990), 15 out of 18 published reports indicated that users of unopposed oestrogens reduced their rate of cardiovascular disease by 50% or more relative to non-users. A more recent quantitative review by Stampfer and Colditz (1991) found a summary relative risk of 0.50 (95% confidence interval 0.43–0.56) for coronary heart disease among women receiving oestrogens relative to non-users for prospective cohort and angiographic studies. Thus, the weight of the evidence suggests that unopposed oestrogens are protective against heart disease. The analyses presented here assumed a 50% decrease in ischaemic heart disease deaths for women receiving unopposed oestrogen. The benefit was assumed to persist for the duration of treatment. Baseline probability of death from ischaemic heart disease was derived from 1983 US life tables.

The evidence concerning the relationship between oestrogen combined with progestin and heart disease is uncertain. Because progestins lower high density lipoprotein (HDL) levels as shown by Ottosson et al (1985) and Wahl et al (1983), which are raised by oestrogens, it is possible that combined hormone replacement therapy will not be as effective in reducing the risk of heart disease as unopposed oestrogen. Therefore, no benefit was assumed for women receiving oestrogen combined with progestin.

Breast cancer

The association between postmenopausal hormone replacement therapy and breast cancer incidence is controversial. Brinton's (1990) recent review of the literature on this topic showed relative risks ranging from 1.5 to 2.1 for various long-term oestrogen treatment durations of at least 5 years. A subsequent report by Colditz et al (1990) found an elevated risk of breast cancer of 1.36 among current users of oestrogen replacement therapy. However, no association was found with the duration of use, suggesting that the increase in risk among current users does not persist following termination of therapy. To reflect these recent data we modelled an increased risk of breast cancer of 1.36 among current users of oestrogens for 2 or more years and assumed that the excess risk would persist for 2 years after the termination of therapy. All other assumptions regarding breast cancer incidence and case fatality rates followed those of Weinstein and Schiff (1982).

Very few studies address the association between oestrogens combined with progestin and the risk of breast cancer. Although a Swedish study by Bergkvist et al (1989) showed an elevated relative risk for long-term users of combined therapy, it did not have adequate power to detect a significant association. As indicated by Barrett-Conner (1989), these results contradict an earlier study by Gambrell (1983), which showed a decreased risk of breast cancer in users of combined oestrogen-progestin therapy. For users of oestrogen combined with progestin, we assumed that the breast cancer risk was not elevated. In separate analyses, however, we allowed for a positive association using the same assumptions as outlined above for users of unopposed oestrogen.

Other event rates

In addition to hip fracture and its sequelae, ischaemic heart disease and breast cancer, our analysis kept account of annual long-term placement in a nursing home for causes other than hip fracture. A report by Cohen et al (1986), which reported data relevant to the age-specific probability of admission to a nursing home for all causes, was used to determine the probability of admission for causes other than hip fracture. Annual probabilities of death from other causes were derived from 1983 US life tables.

Costs

All costs are represented in 1990 US dollars. Hip fracture costs ranged from $12 810 at 50–59 years of age to $15 125 at 80–89 years of age. These figures included hospital costs as estimated from Medicare data, and surgeons' and other professional fees as described by Tosteson et al (1990).

Based on Medicare data, Eddy (1989) reported that the Division of Cancer Prevention and Control of the National Cancer Institute estimated a charge of approximately $7970 for non-invasive breast cancers. We used this figure, which does not include the cost of terminal care, to estimate the cost of an incident case of breast cancer.

The cost of hormone replacement therapy was $193 per year for un-opposed oestrogen and $250 per year for oestrogen-progestin therapy. These costs are assumed to include any extra physician visits that are required for treatment and monitoring. To estimate the cost of nursing home residency, the average per day rate for skilled nursing homes as reported by the National Center for Health Statistics (1987) was used. Thus, nursing home residency was estimated to cost approximately $31 940 per year.

Quality of life

Although there are many approaches to the elicitation of patient preferences from which quality weights are derived, one approach is to determine the proportion of a year of life in perfect health that a patient would be willing to trade for a year of life in her current health state. Thus the quality weights that are assigned to each health state in the Markov model represent the fraction of a year in perfect health that is equivalent to 1 year in the impaired health state. For example, a patient living in a nursing home who would be willing to exchange 1 year in the nursing home for 0.4 years in perfect health (residing outside of the nursing home) would have a quality weight of 0.4 assigned to the nursing home health state. To compute quality-adjusted life expectancy, we adopted the quality weights used by Hillner et al (1986) in their evaluation of oestrogen replacement therapy. The quality weights for acute hip fracture states were as follows: 0.95 for an uncomplicated hip fracture, 0.76 for a disabling hip fracture and 0.36 for a hip fracture that required nursing home placement. The quality weights for long-term disability and nursing home residency were 0.8 and 0.4, respectively.

HORMONE REPLACEMENT THERAPY RELATIVE TO NO INTERVENTION

Impact on cost

For all hormone replacement regimens, the total discounted cost of treatment outweighed the total discounted savings from decreased hip fracture incidence and nursing home residency (Table 2). Savings from hip fracture range from \$315 to \$435 and savings from decreased nursing home utilization, which are more than twice as great, range from \$675 to \$903. The increase in total expected costs from increased breast cancer incidence are

Table 2. Components of total expected discounted costs in 1990 US dollars for an individual patient age 50 years receiving hormone replacement therapy relative to an individual receiving no treatment. The changes in total expected cost (dC) that reflect the baseline assumptions for each hormone replacement regimen are given in bold. Components represent the cost of hormone replacement therapy (dC_{HRT}), savings from decreased hip fracture incidence (dC_{HFX}), savings from decreased nursing home residency (dC_{NH}), and costs from increased breast cancer incidence (dC_{BRCA}). E-10 represents 10 years of oestrogen therapy, E-15 represents 15 years of oestrogen therapy, EP-10 represents 10 years of oestrogen-progestin therapy and EP-15 represents 15 years of oestrogen-progestin therapy.

| | Hormone replacement therapy regimen | | | |
| | Previous hysterectomy | | Uterus intact | |
Component	E-10	E-15	EP-10	EP-15
dC_{HRT}	\$1532	\$2031	\$1990	\$2638
dC_{HFX}	−315	−435	−315	−435
dC_{NH}	−675	−903	−675	−903
dC_{BRCA}	36	52	36	52
Totals				
$dC_{HRT+HFX}$	\$1217	\$1596	\$1675	\$2203
$dC_{HRT+HFX+NH}$	542	693	**1000**	**1300**
$dC_{HRT+HFX+NH+BRCA}$	**578**	**745**	1036	1352

small relative to the costs of therapy. We did not model incident cases of ischaemic heart disease and thus were unable to estimate the expected savings per person treated with hormone replacement therapy that would result from a reduction in ischaemic heart disease incidence. If this unknown component of savings were to exceed \$578 or \$745 for the 10- and 15-year oestrogen regimens, respectively, then treatment with hormone replacement therapy would be cost-saving relative to no intervention. Likewise, if combined therapy were to confer a benefit in decreased ischaemic heart disease incidence, oestrogen-progestin therapy would become cost-saving if the savings associated with heart disease were to exceed \$1036 or \$1352 for 10- and 15-year durations, respectively.

Impact on life expectancy

The individual gains in life expectancy from decreased hip fracture incidence for hormone replacement therapy relative to no therapy range from 0.0519 to 0.0732 years (19 to 27 days) (Table 3). When an increased risk of breast cancer was modelled, the losses in life expectancy, which ranged from 0.0401 to 0.0577 years (15 to 21 days), almost eliminated the gains from decreased hip fracture incidence. The largest gain in life expectancy was from the decrease in ischaemic heart disease death, which ranged from 0.0597 to 0.2235 years (22 to 82 days) depending on the duration of treatment and the assumption regarding reduction in risk of death from ischaemic heart disease that was modelled. These findings are consistent with reports by Henderson et al (1988) and Hillner et al (1986), which indicate that any reduction in heart disease that is associated with hormone replacement therapy will overwhelm all other components of the risk-benefit equation. They are also consistent with the estimate of Cummings et al (1989) that the lifetime risk of death from heart disease is 10 times greater than the risk of death from either hip fracture or breast cancer.

Table 3. Components of change in total undiscounted (part A) and discounted (part B) life expectancy are expressed in years for an individual patient aged 50 years receiving hormone replacement therapy relative to an individual receiving no treatment. The changes in life expectancy (dLE) that reflect the baseline assumptions for each hormone replacement regimen are given in bold. The components represent the gain from decreased hip fracture incidence (dLE_{HFX}), losses from increased breast cancer incidence (dLE_{BRCA}), gains from decreased ischaemic heart disease deaths under the assumption that deaths are reduced by 25% (dLE_{IHD-75}) or 50% (dLE_{IHD-50}) in users of hormone replacement therapy relative to non-users. E-10 represents 10 years of oestrogen therapy, E-15 represents 15 years of oestrogen therapy, EP-10 represents 10 years of oestrogen-progestin therapy and EP-15 represents 15 years of oestrogen-progestin therapy.

| | Hormone replacement therapy regimen | | | |
| | Previous hysterectomy | | Uterus intact | |
Component	E-10	E-15	EP-10	EP-15
Part A: Undiscounted life expectancy				
dLE_{HFX}	0.0519	0.0732	0.0519	0.0732
dLE_{BRCA}	−0.0401	−0.0577	−0.0401	−0.0577
dLE_{IHD-75}	0.0597	0.1115	0.0597	0.1115
dLE_{IHD-50}	0.1140	0.2235	0.1140	0.2235
Totals				
$dLE_{HFX\ only}$	0.0519	0.0732	**0.0519**	**0.0732**
$dLE_{HFX+BRCA}$	0.0118	0.0155	0.0118	0.0155
$dLE_{HFX+BRCA+IHD-50}$	**0.1258**	**0.2390**	0.1258	0.2390
Part B: Discounted life expectancy				
dLE_{HFX}	0.0113	0.0151	0.0113	0.0151
dLE_{BRCA}	−0.0108	−0.0133	−0.0108	−0.0133
dLE_{IHD-75}	0.0226	0.0399	0.0226	0.0399
dLE_{IHD-50}	0.0453	0.0798	0.0453	0.0798
Totals				
$dLE_{HFX\ only}$	0.0113	0.0151	**0.0113**	**0.0151**
$dLE_{HFX+BRCA}$	0.0005	0.0018	0.0005	0.0018
$dLE_{HFX+BRCA+IHD-50}$	**0.0458**	**0.0816**	0.0458	0.0816

Impact on quality of life

When quality of life was considered, decreased hip fracture incidence accounted for additional gains of between 0.0647 and 0.0881 quality-adjusted years (24 and 32 days) (Table 4). Included in this component of quality of life are the decreases in disability, acute morbidity and nursing home utilization that are associated with hip fracture. If hormone replacement therapy were to reduce quality of life by between 0.4 and 1.8 days per year of therapy ($dQ_{SYMPT:0.999}$ to $dQ_{SYMPT:0.995}$), then losses in overall quality of life for the hormone replacement therapy regimens would range from 0.0096 to 0.0712 years (4 to 26 days). When the differential timing of events is taken into account in the discounted analysis, reductions in quality of life of 1.1 days ($dQ_{SYMPT:0.997}$) or more per year quickly outweigh the gains achieved from decreased hip fracture incidence and its sequelae (Table 4). Thus, individual patient preference regarding use of

Table 4. Components of change in total discounted (part A) and undiscounted (part B) quality-adjusted life years for an individual patient aged 50 years receiving hormone replacement therapy relative to an individual receiving no treatment. Components represent gains in quality-adjusted life years from decreased hip fracture incidence, disability and long-term nursing home residency (dQ_{HFX}) and losses from symptoms associated with hormone replacement therapy under the assumption that 1 year of therapy is equivalent to 0.999, 0.997 or 0.995 years without therapy ($dQ_{SYMPT:0.999}$, $dQ_{SYMPT:0.997}$ and $dQ_{SYMPT:0.995}$, respectively). E-10 represents 10 years of oestrogen therapy, E-15 represents 15 years of oestrogen therapy, EP-10 represents 10 years of oestrogen-progestin therapy and EP-15 represents 15 years of oestrogen-progestin therapy.

| | Hormone replacement therapy regimen | | | |
| | Previous hysterectomy | | Uterus intact | |
Component	E-10	E-15	EP-10	EP-15
Part A: Undiscounted quality-adjusted life years				
dQ_{HFX}	0.0647	0.0881	0.0647	0.0881
$dQ_{SYMPT:0.999}$	−0.0096	−0.0142	−0.0096	−0.0142
$dQ_{SYMPT:0.997}$	−0.0292	−0.0427	−0.0292	−0.0427
$dQ_{SYMPT:0.995}$	−0.0486	−0.0712	−0.0486	−0.0712
Totals				
dQ_{HFX}	0.0647	0.0881	0.0647	0.0881
$dQ_{HFX+SYMPT:0.999}$	0.0551	0.0739	0.0551	0.0551
$dQ_{HFX+SYMPT:0.997}$	0.0355	0.0454	0.0355	0.0454
$dQ_{HFX+SYMPT:0.995}$	0.0161	0.0169	0.0161	0.0169
Part B: Discounted quality-adjusted life years				
dQ_{HFX}	0.0183	0.0247	0.0183	0.0247
$dQ_{SYMPT:0.999}$	−0.0085	−0.0104	−0.0085	−0.0104
$dQ_{SYMPT:0.997}$	−0.0254	−0.0313	−0.0254	−0.0313
$dQ_{SYMPT:0.995}$	−0.0424	−0.0522	−0.0424	−0.0522
Totals				
dQ_{HFX}	0.0183	0.0247	0.0183	0.0247
$dQ_{HFX+SYMPT:0.999}$	0.0098	0.0143	0.0098	0.0143
$dQ_{HFX+SYMPT:0.997}$	−0.0071	−0.0066	−0.0071	−0.0066
$dQ_{HFX+SYMPT:0.995}$	−0.0241	−0.0275	−0.0241	−0.0275

hormone replacement therapy and its side-effects are important for the assessment of quality of life.

Quality-adjusted life expectancy

Components of life expectancy and quality-adjusted life expectancy were combined to estimate quality-adjusted life expectancy for various treatment regimens and assumptions (Table 5). Depending on the components included in the computation, overall gains in quality-adjusted life expectancy ranged from 0.0473 to 0.3271 years (17 to 119 days). In the discounted analysis, however, when ischaemic heart disease was excluded

Table 5. Change in total undiscounted (part A) and discounted (part B) quality-adjusted life expectancy for an individual patient aged 50 years receiving hormone replacement therapy relative to no therapy when various components of life expectancy and quality are considered. E-10 represents 10 years of oestrogen therapy, E-15 represents 15 years of oestrogen therapy, EP-10 represents 10 years of oestrogen-progestin therapy and EP-15 represents 15 years of oestrogen-progestin therapy.

| | Hormone replacement therapy regimen | | | |
| | Previous hysterectomy | | Uterus intact | |
$dQALE$	E-10	E-15	EP-10	EP-15
Part A: Undiscounted quality-adjusted life expectancy				
$dLE_{HFX}+dQ_{HFX}$	0.1166	0.1613	0.1166	0.1613
$dLE_{HFX+BRCA}+dQ_{HFX}$	0.0765	0.1036	0.0765	0.1036
$dLE_{HFX+BRCA}+dQ_{HFX+SYMPT:0.997}$	0.0473	0.0609	0.0473	0.0609
$dLE_{HFX+BRCA+IHD-50}+dQ_{HFX}$	0.1905	0.3271	0.1905	0.3271
$dLE_{HFX+BRCA+IHD-50}+dQ_{HFX+SYMPT:0.997}$	0.1613	0.2844	0.1613	0.2844
Part B: Discounted quality-adjusted life expectancy				
$dLE_{HFX}+dQ_{HFX}$	0.0296	0.0398	0.0296	0.0398
$dLE_{HFX+BRCA}+dQ_{HFX}$	0.0188	0.0265	0.0188	0.0265
$dLE_{HFX+BRCA}+dQ_{HFX+SYMPT:0.997}$	−0.0066	−0.0048	−0.0066	−0.0048
$dLE_{HFX+BRCA+IHD-50}+dQ_{HFX}$	0.0641	0.1063	0.0641	0.1063
$dLE_{HFX+BRCA+IHD-50}+dQ_{HFX+SYMPT:0.997}$	0.0387	0.0750	0.0387	0.0750

from the risk-benefit equation and hormone replacement therapy was assumed to decrease quality of life by 1.1 days per year ($dQ_{SYMPT:0.997}$), all forms of treatment resulted in an overall loss in quality-adjusted life expectancy relative to no intervention.

Cost-effectiveness of hormone replacement

The cost-effectiveness ratios were previously defined as additional cost per year of life saved (dC/dLE) and additional cost per quality-adjusted year of life saved ($dC/dQALE$). Using the discounted components of change in cost (Table 2), life-expectancy (Table 3) and quality-adjusted life expectancy (Table 5), these ratios can be formed for each treatment regimen under a variety of assumptions.

Under the baseline assumptions for unopposed oestrogen therapy (Table 6), which include an increased risk of breast cancer (36%) and a decreased risk of ischaemic heart disease death (50%), the additional cost per year of life saved for a 10-year course of therapy relative to no intervention is $12 620. For a 15-year course of unopposed oestrogen, the cost is $9130 per year of life saved. These results apply only to women with a prior hysterectomy, which is the only group for which unopposed oestrogen replacement was considered.

Under the baseline assumptions for combined oestrogen-progestin therapy (Table 6), which includes no increased risk of breast cancer or decreased risk of ischaemic heart disease death, the additional cost per year of life saved for a 10-year course of therapy is $88 500. For a 15-year course of combined therapy, the cost is $86 100 per year of life saved.

When quality of life adjustments were made for hip fracture and its sequelae, the costs per year of life saved for oestrogen in women with a prior hysterectomy decreased to $9020 and $7010 for 10- and 15-year treatment durations, respectively. The costs per quality-adjusted year of life saved for combined therapy in women with an intact uterus were $33 780 and $32 660

Table 6. Summary of baseline assumptions concerning increased (↑), decreased (↓), or unchanged (→) risks of hormone replacement therapy. E-10 represents 10 years of oestrogen therapy, E-15 represents 15 years of oestrogen therapy, EP-10 represents 10 years of oestrogen-progestin therapy and EP-15 represents 15 years of oestrogen-progestin therapy.

| | Hormone replacement therapy regimen | | | |
| | Previous hysterectomy | | Uterus intact | |
Risk/benefit	E-10	E-15	EP-10	EP-15
Hip fracture incidence	↓	↓	↓	↓
Breast cancer incidence	↑ 36%	↑ 36%	→	→
Ischaemic heart disease death	↓ 50%	↓ 50%	→	→

for 10- and 15-year treatment durations, respectively. When an additional adjustment in quality of life of -1.1 days per year ($dQ_{SYMPT:0.997}$) for hormone replacement therapy was considered, the ratios for unopposed oestrogen increased slightly to $14 940 and $9930 per quality-adjusted year of life saved. When the additional adjustment was made for combined oestrogen-progestin therapy, however, the cost per quality-adjusted year of life saved jumped to over $150 000 for both treatment durations.

If oestrogen-progestin therapy were to confer an increased risk of breast cancer, without decreasing the risk of ischaemic heart disease death, the costs per year of life saved for 10- and 15-year regimens would exceed $700 000. Likewise, if oestrogen conferred an increased risk of breast cancer, without decreasing the risk of death from ischaemic heart disease, the costs per year of life saved for 10- and 15-year regimens would also increase, with both ratios exceeding $400 000.

Under baseline assumptions, the ratios that were estimated for unopposed oestrogen in women with a prior hysterectomy compare very favourably with the cost-effectiveness of other commonly accepted medical practices. For example, Weinstein and Stason (1985) estimated that the treatment of mild diastolic hypertension cost $25 000 per quality-adjusted year of life gained and coronary artery bypass surgery in patients with three vessel disease cost approximately $6000 per year of life gained. Furthermore, it is important to note that no savings associated with the decrease in ischaemic heart disease mortality (and presumably incidence) were included in the computation of cost-effectiveness. It is possible that savings from ischaemic heart disease would overwhelm the costs of hormone replacement therapy, making it cost-saving relative to no intervention. In contrast to unopposed oestrogen for women with a prior hysterectomy, combined therapy appears more costly, with ratios in excess of $145 000 per year of life saved. The difference between the cost-effectiveness of unopposed oestrogen and oestrogen-progestin is attributable to the inclusion of decreased ischaemic heart disease deaths in the risk-benefit equation for unopposed oestrogen. Further research is needed to determine the impact of combined therapy on ischaemic heart disease incidence and death.

HORMONE REPLACEMENT THERAPY RELATIVE TO SCREENING

Although hormone replacement therapy is clearly cost-effective when compared with other medical practices under the assumption that it decreases ischaemic heart disease deaths by 50%, we have observed how costly therapy is when heart disease deaths are not considered. We therefore consider alternative oestrogen-progestin treatment regimens, which involve screening perimenopausal women using dual-photon absorptiometry of the hip and selectively treating only those women who are judged to be at risk of hip fracture on the basis of their bone density measurement.

For a 15-year treatment duration, Tosteson et al (1990) reported incremental cost-effectiveness ratios for screening strategies ranging from $11 700 to $94 700 in 1987 US dollars. In comparison to the most aggressive screening strategy, which would treat 61.2% of the population, unselective hormone replacement therapy was found to cost an additional $349 000 per year of life saved. Although strategies were more cost-effective when quality of life was considered, the additional cost of unselective treatment remained well above $100 000 per additional year of life saved.

When an increased risk of breast cancer was assumed for women receiving oestrogen-progestin therapy for 2 or more years until 2 years following termination of therapy, the argument in favour of screening is strengthened. Inflating the results of Tosteson et al (1990) to 1990 US dollars and combining them with our current estimates of decrease in life expectancy (dLE_{BRCA}) and increase in cost (dC_{BRCA}) from breast cancer, we found that only the screening strategy that instituted treatment at bone mineral densities below $0.9 \, g/cm^2$ had a ratio below $50 000 per additional year of life saved. Unselective treatment and treating at a threshold of less than $1.1 \, g/cm^2$ resulted in a net decrease in life expectancy.

Melton et al (1990) discussed the clinical indications for bone mass measurement and concluded that unselective screening for osteoporosis could not be recommended until further data are available. As noted by

Tosteson et al (1990), because our underlying model's relative risks for hip fracture at ages 60 and 80 for a patient entering the model with a bone density of 1 standard deviation below the mean bone mineral density at age 50 years were higher than estimates from prospective studies by Cummings et al (1990) and Hui et al (1989), further prospective data are required before widespread cost-effective screening guidelines can be established. However, if ongoing prospective studies validate the underlying risks of hip fracture with the decreasing bone mineral density that our estimates are based on, and if oestrogen-progestin therapy confers no benefit with respect to heart disease, the most cost-effective clinical management strategy may involve bone mineral density screening for women with an intact uterus. Under this scenario, the consideration of screening strategies would become even more important when breast cancer is modelled as a risk of therapy or when decrements in quality of life are included for women receiving combined therapy.

LIMITATIONS

This analysis has estimated the cost-effectiveness of hormone replacement therapy in two populations of perimenopausal women. We emphasize that we have not compared the cost-effectiveness of unopposed oestrogen with the cost-effectiveness of combined oestrogen-progestin therapy for women with an intact uterus. Such a comparison would require that endometrial monitoring, hyperplasia and cancer be included in both the risk-benefit and cost components of the cost-effectiveness ratio.

This analysis did not consider the occurrence of other osteoporotic fractures of the wrist and vertebrae, which are common in postmenopausal women. Although these fractures are not associated with the high excess mortality of hip fracture, they are associated with a high degree of morbidity and warrant consideration. The large impact that fractures of the wrist and vertebrae are likely to have on quality-adjusted life expectancy would favourably affect the cost-effectiveness ratios for hormone replacement therapy when added to the risk-benefit equation.

Another issue that merits consideration is the cost-effectiveness of hormone replacement in elderly postmenopausal women. Resnick and Greenspan (1989) have reviewed the issues that pertain to osteoporosis in women over the age of 70. Because women in this age range have already lost substantial amounts of bone, it is not clear how much benefit from decreased incidence of osteoporotic fractures would be achieved by treating this population with hormone replacement therapy.

SUMMARY

The net resource costs and net health benefits of treating perimenopausal women with hormone replacement therapy were evaluated within the framework of cost-effectiveness analysis. Data from the epidemiological literature were used to estimate changes in discounted life expectancy from hip fracture, ischaemic heart disease and breast cancer that are associated with hormone replacement therapy under a variety of assumptions. Economic data were used to estimate changes in total discounted costs that result from the use of hormone replacement therapy. For women with a previous hysterectomy, 10- and 15-year courses of unopposed oestrogen were evaluated. The baseline assumptions for unopposed oestrogen were that breast cancer incidence would be increased for current users by 36% and that deaths from ischaemic heart disease would be reduced by 50% relative to non-users. Under these assumptions, oestrogen replacement therapy was found to be cost-effective, with ratios ranging from $9130 to $12 620 per additional year of life saved. For women who have not had a hysterectomy, 10- and 15-year courses of oestrogen combined with pro-gestin were evaluated. The baseline assumptions for combined therapy were that breast cancer incidence and ischaemic heart disease deaths were unaffected. Under these assumptions, combined therapy was more costly, with ratios ranging from $86 100 to $88 500. Unless combined therapy is found to confer protection against ischaemic heart disease, the most cost-effective strategies for women with no prior hysterectomy may involve screening perimenopausal women to detect women at highest risk of hip fracture followed by selective treatment.

REFERENCES

Barrett-Conner E (1989) Postmenopausal estrogen replacement and breast cancer. *New England Journal of Medicine* **321**: 319–320.

Beck JR & Pauker SG (1983) The Markov model of medical prognosis. *Medical Decision Making* **3**: 419–458.

Bergkvist L, Adami H, Persson I, Hoover R & Schairer C (1989) The risk of breast cancer after estrogen and estrogen-progestin replacement. *New England Journal of Medicine* **321**: 293–297.

Brinton LA (1990) Menopause and the risk of breast cancer. *Annals of the New York Academy of Sciences* **592**: 357–362.

Bush TL (1990) The epidemiology of cardiovascular disease in postmenopausal women. *Annals of the New York Academy of Sciences* **592**: 263–271.

Christiansen C, Christensen MS & Transbol I (1981) Bone mass in postmenopausal women after withdrawal of oestrogen/gestagen replacement therapy. *Lancet* **i**: 459–461.

Cohen MA, Tell EJ & Wallack SS (1986) The lifetime risks and costs of nursing home use among the elderly. *Medical Care* **24**: 1161–1172.

Colditz GA, Stampfer MJ, Willet WC, Hennekens CH, Rosner B & Speizer FE (1990) Prospective study of estrogen replacement therapy and risk of breast cancer in post-menopausal women. *Journal of the American Medical Association* **264**: 2648–2653.

Cummings SR, Black DM & Rubin SM (1989) Lifetime risks of hip, Colles', or vertebral fracture and coronary heart disease among white postmenopausal women. *Archives of Internal Medicine* **149**: 2445–2448.

Cummings SR, Black DM, Nevitt MC et al: Study of Osteoporotic Fractures Research Group (1990) Appendicular bone density and age predict hip fracture in women. *Journal of the American Medical Association* **263**: 665–668.

Dahl E (1980) Mortality and life expectancy after hip fractures. *Acta Orthopaedica Scandinavica* **51**: 163–170.

Eddy DM (1989) Screening for breast cancer. *Annals of Internal Medicine* **111**: 389–399.

Eisenberg JM (1989) Clinical economics: A guide to the economic analysis of clinical practices. *Journal of the American Medical Association* **262**: 2879–2886.

Ettinger B, Genant HK & Cann CE (1985) Long-term estrogen replacement therapy prevents bone loss and fractures. *Annals of Internal Medicine* **102**: 319–324.

Gambrell RD Jr, Maier RC & Sanders BI (1983) Decreased incidence of breast cancer in postmenopausal estrogen-progestogen users. *Obstetrics and Gynecology* **62**: 435–443.

Henderson BE, Ross RK, Lobo RA, Pike MC & Mack TM (1988) Re-evaluating the role of progestogen therapy after the menopause. *Fertility and Sterility* **49(Supplement)**: 9S–15S.

Hillner BE, Hollenberg JP & Pauker SG (1986) Postmenopausal estrogens in prevention of osteoporosis: Benefit virtually without risk if cardiovascular effects are considered. *American Journal of Medicine* **80**: 1115–1117.

Hui SL, Slemenda CW & Johnston CC (1989) Baseline measurement of bone mass predicts fracture in white women. *Annals of Internal Medicine* **111**: 355–361.

Kenzora JE, McCarthy RE, Lowell JD & Sledge CB (1984) Hip fracture mortality: Relation to age, treatment, preoperative illness, time of surgery, and complications. *Clinical Orthopaedics and Related Research* **186**: 45–56.

Kiel DP, Felson DT, Anderson JJ, Wilson PWF & Moskowitz MA (1987) Hip fracture and the use of estrogens in postmenopausal women: The Framingham study. *New England Journal of Medicine* **317**: 1169–1174.

Kreutzfeld J, Haim M & Bach E (1984) Hip fracture among the elderly in a mixed urban and rural population. *Age and Ageing* **13**: 111–119.

Lindsay R, Hart DM, MacLean A, Clarke AC, Kraszewski A & Garwood J (1978) Bone response to termination of oestrogen treatment. *Lancet* **i**: 1325–1327.

Melton LJ III, Wahner HW, Richelson LS, O'Fallon WM & Riggs BL (1986) Osteoporosis and the risk of hip fracture. *American Journal of Epidemiology* **124**: 254–261.

Melton LJ, Kan SH, Wahner HW & Riggs BL (1988) Lifetime fracture risk: An approach to hip fracture risk assessment based on bone mineral density and age. *Journal of Clinical Epidemiology* **41**: 985–994.

Melton LJ, Eddy DM & Johnston CC (1990) Screening for osteoporosis. *Annals of Internal Medicine* **112**: 516–528.

Miller CW (1978) Survival and ambulation following hip fracture. *Journal of Bone and Joint Surgery* **7**: 930–934.

Mossey JM, Mutran E, Knott K & Craik R (1989) Determinants of recovery 12 months after hip fracture: The importance of psychosocial factors. *American Journal of Public Health* **79**: 279–286.

National Center for Health Statistics (1987) Use of nursing homes by the elderly: Preliminary data from the 1985 National Nursing Home Survey. *Advance Data From Vital and Health Statistics*, no. 135 (DHHS publication no. (PHS)87-1250). Hyattsville, Maryland: US Public Health Service.

Ottosson UB, Johansson BG & von Schoultz B (1985) Subfractions of high-density lipoprotein cholesterol during estrogen replacement therapy: A comparison between progestogens and natural progesterone. *American Journal of Obstetrics and Gynecology* **151**: 745–750.

Persson I, Adami H, Bergkvist L et al (1989) Risk of endometrial cancer after treatment with oestrogens alone or in conjunction with progestogens: results of a prospective study. *British Medical Journal* **298**: 147–151.

Pettiti DB & Sidney S (1989) Hip fracture in women: Incidence, in-hospital mortality and five-year survival probabilities in members of a pre-paid health plan. *Clinical Orthopaedics and Related Research* **246**: 150–155.

Quigley MET, Martin PL, Burnier AM & Brooks P (1987) Estrogen therapy arrests bone loss in elderly women. *American Journal of Obstetrics and Gynecology* **156**: 1516–1523.

Resnick NM & Greenspan SL (1989) 'Senile' osteoporosis reconsidered. *Journal of the American Medical Association* **261**: 1025–1029.

Stampfer MJ & Colditz GA (1991) Estrogen replacement therapy and coronary heart disease: A quantitative assessment of the epidemiologic evidence. *Preventive Medicine* **20**: 47–63.

Tosteson ANA, Rosenthal DI, Melton LJ III & Weinstein MC (1990) Cost effectiveness of screening perimenopausal white women for osteoporosis: Bone densitometry and hormone replacement therapy. *Annals of Internal Medicine* **113**: 594–603.

US Preventive Services Task Force (1990) Estrogen prophylaxis. *American Family Physician* **42**: 1293–1296.

Utian WH (1988) Consensus statement on progestin use in postmenopausal women. *Maturitas* **11:** 175–177.

Wahl P, Walden C, Knopp R et al (1983) Effect of estrogen/progestin potency on lipid/lipoprotein cholesterol. *New England Journal of Medicine* **308:** 862–867.

Weinstein MC (1980) Estrogen use in postmenopausal women—costs, risks, and benefits. *New England Journal of Medicine* **303:** 308–316.

Weinstein MC & Schiff I (1982) Cost-effectiveness of hormone replacement therapy in the menopause. *Obstetrical and Gynecological Survey* **38:** 445–455.

Weinstein MC & Stason WB (1977) Foundations of cost-effectiveness analysis for health and medical practices. *New England Journal of Medicine* **296:** 716–721.

Weinstein MC & Stason WB (1985) Cost-effectiveness of interventions to prevent or treat coronary heart disease. *Annual Review of Public Health* **6:** 41–63.

Weinstein MC & Tosteson ANA (1990) Cost-effectiveness of hormone replacement. *Annals of the New York Academy of Sciences* **592:** 162–172.

Weiss NS, Ure CL, Ballard JH, Williams AR & Daling JR (1980) Decreased risk of fractures of the hip and lower forearm with postmenopausal use of estrogens. *New England Journal of Medicine* **303:** 1195–1198.

Weiss NS, Liff JM, Ure CL, Ballard JH, Abbott GH & Daling JR (1983) Mortality in women following hip fracture. *Journal of Chronic Diseases* **36:** 879–882.

Ziel HK (1982) Estrogen's role in endometrial cancer. *Obstetrics and Gynecology* **60:** 509–515.

Index

Note: Page numbers of article titles are in **bold** type.

Absorptiometry, 808–810
  dual energy X-ray, 810
  dual photon, 809–810
  single photon, 808–809
Acid phosphatase, 821–822
Age—
  morbidity and, 797–798
  -related bone loss, 792–794
Aldendronate, 860–861
Alkaline phosphatase, 818–819
Anabolic steroids, 863
Atherosclerosis, *see* Coronary atherosclerosis
  and also Heart disease

BGP, *see* Osteocalcin
Biochemical bone markers, **817–830, 831–836**
Bisphosphonates, 860–861
Blood clotting, 822, 893
Bone formation stimulation, 862–864
Bone gla protein, *see* Osteocalcin
Bone loss, and menopause, *see under* Menopause *and also* Osteoporosis
Bone markers, *see* Biochemical bone markers
Bone mass, 832–833
  peak, 791–792
Bone mass measurements, 795–796, **807–815**
  techniques of, 808–811
    dual energy X-ray absorptiometry, 810
    dual photon absorptiometry, 809–810
    quantitative CT, 810–811
    radiogrammetry, 808
    single photon absorptiometry, 809–810
Bone mineral content, **853–856**
  see also Bone mass measurements
Bone mineral density, 795–796
  see also Bone mass measurements
Bone resorption inhibition, 859–862
Bone resorption markers, *see* Biochemical bone markers
Bone sialoprotein II (BSP), 820
Bone turnover—
  at menopause, 823–825
  hip fracture, 826
  vertebral osteoporosis and, 825–826

in the monkey, 923–926
Breast cancer, 948
  and oestrogen therapy, 895–897

Calcitonin, 860
Calcitriol, 861
Calcium—
  dietary, 847–848
  metabolism, 831–832
  therapeutic, 859–860
Cancer, and oestrogen replacement therapy, 893–897
  breast, 895–897, 948
  endometrial, 894–895
γ-Carboxyglutamic acid, 822
Cardiovascular disease, *see* Heart disease
Clodronate, 861
Clotting factors, 822
  oestrogen therapy and, 893
Collagen, 831–832
Collagen I, 819–820
Collagen pyridinium crosslinks, 822–823
Computed tomography, *see* Quantitative CT
Coronary atherosclerosis, monkey, **915–934**
Coronary heart disease, *see* Heart disease
Cost-effectiveness ratios, 945
Cost, of osteoporotic fractures, 799–800
CVD, *see* Heart disease
Cynomolgus macaques, *see under* Coronary atherosclerosis, monkey
Cyproterone acetate, 874–882

Deoxypyridinoline, 822–823, 832
DEXA, *see* Dual energy X-ray absorptiometry
Diethylstilbestrol, 894
1,25-Dihydroxycholecalciferol, 861–862
Disability, and osteoporosis, 799
Distal forearm fractures, *see* Fractures
Dual photon absorptiometry, 809–810, 923
Dual energy X-ray absorptiometry, 810, 925
Dydrogestrone, 874–882

Endometrial cancer, and oestrogen therapy, 894–895

Enzyme markers, 818–823
Estraderm, 846, 891
Ethinyloestradiol, 921–922
Etidronate, 860–861
Exercise, 848, 863

Fluoride, 862
Fractures, 788, **935–942**, 946–947
    consequences of, 939–940
    hip, 826, 946–947
    incidence of, 936–937, 940–941
    prediction of, 796–797
    prevention risk, 936
    research, 941
    risk factors, 936–938
    skeletal fragility and, 785–788
    vertebral osteoporosis and, 825–826

Galactosyl hydrolysine, 821
Glycosides, hydroxylysine, 821
Growth factors, 863–864

HDL, *see under* Lipoproteins
Heart disease, 867–869, **915–934**, 947–948
    and oestrogen replacement therapy, 897–
        908
    and oestrogen therapy, **889–913**
    post-menopausal, HRT and, 881–882
Hepatic metabolism, oestrogen therapy and,
    892–893
Hip fracture, 826, 946–947
    see also Fractures
Hormone replacement therapy (HRT), 853–
        856, 881–882, **943–959**
    and no-intervention therapy, 950–955
    oestrogen, 890–908
    regimes for, 943–944
    screening, 955–956
    state transition, Markov, 945–946
    using cost-effectiveness principles, 944–
        945, 949–950, 953–956
        net health benefit, 944
        net resource, 945
        ratios, 945
Hot flush, 891
Hydroxylysine glycosides, 821
Hydroxyllysylpyridinoline, 822–823
17-Hydroxyprogesterones, 880–881
Hydroxyproline, 820–821

125I, 808–809
Intertrochanteric fracture, 788–790
Intramuscular oestrogens, 873

LDL, *see* Lipoproteins
Levonorgestrel, 874–882
Life expectancy, and HRT, 950–951
    quality-adjusted, 953
Lipids, *see under* Lipoproteins

Lipoproteins, **867–887**
    and the contraceptive steroid effect, 918–
        922
    heart disease and, 867–869
    HRT and, 881–882
    menopause and, 869–871
    oestrogen therapy and, 871–874
        and progestogens, 874–881
    ovarian function, monkey, 916–917
    pregnancy, in the monkey, 917–918
    sex differences, in the monkey, 915–916
Liver, and oestrogen therapy, 892–893
Lynoestrenol, 874–882
Lysylpyridinoline, 822–823

Markov state-transition models, 945–946
Medroxyprogesterone acetate, 846–847, 874–
    882
Megestrol acetate, 874–882
Menopause, 837–843
    bone loss, 794
    bone turnover, 823–825
    lipoprotein, 869–871
    in the monkey, **915–934**
    and oestrogen replacement, 891–892
    post-
        and HRT, 881–882
        vertebral osteoporosis, 825–826
    symptoms, 891–892
Monkeys, and osteoporosis, **915–934**
Morbidity, and osteoporosis, 797–798
Mortality, and osteoporosis, 798–799

Nandrolone decanoate, 863
Net health benefit, 944
Net resource cost, 945
Norethindrone acetate, 853–855, 874–882

Oestradiol, 926–929
Oestrogen-progestins, and HRT cost-
    effectiveness, 948
Oestrogen replacement therapy, 890–908
    cancer, 893–897
    complications, 892–897
    heart disease, 897–908
    indications, 891–892
    liver and, 892–893
    post-menopausal monkey, 926–931
Oestrogens, 843–847, 871–874
    i.m., 873
    oral, 871–872
    parenteral, 890–891, 906–907
    percutaneous, 873–874
    progestogens, 874–881
    s.c., 873
    transdermal, 873–874
    vaginal, 872–873, 890
Oral oestrogens, 871–872, 890
Osteoblasts, and oestrogen, 841–843

Osteocalcin, 819, 831, 841
Osteonectin, 820
Osteoporosis—
  age-related bone loss, 792–794
  bone mass, *see under* Bone mass measurements
  cardiovascular disease, **889–913**
  coronary atherosclerosis, **915–934**
  cost, of fractures, 799–800
  diagnostics, 811–814
  disability, 799
  epidemiology of, **785–805**
  fractures, 788, **935–942**, 946–947
    prediction of, 796–797
  future of epidemiology, 800–801
  HRT and, **853–856**
    post-menopause, 943–959
  menopause, *see* Menopause
  menopausal bone loss, 794
  monkeys and, **915–934**
  morbidity, 797–798
  mortality, 789–799
  oestrogen, and cardiovascular disease, **889–913**
  oestrogens, and coronary atherosclerosis, **915–934**
  pathogenesis of, 785–790
  prevention, **837–852**
  replacement, *see* Oestrogen replacement therapy
  risk factors, 790–795, 832–833
  serum lipids, and sex steroids, 867–887
  and sex steroid alternatives, **857–865**
  skeletal fragility, 785–788
  therapy principles, 857–859
  trauma risk, 788–790

Paget's disease, 817, 822
Parathyroid hormone, 863–864
Parenteral oestrogen, 890–891, 906–907
Peak bone mass, 791–792
Percutaneous oestrogens, 873–874
Phosphatases—
  acid, 821–822
  alkaline, 818–819
Photon absorptiometry, 808–810
  dual, 809–810
  single, 808–809
Plasma tartrate-resistant acid phosphatase, 821–822
Precision, and bone mass measurements, 811–812

Pregnancy, monkey, 917–918
Procollagen I, 819–820
Progestogen-oestrogen combinations, 874–884
  17-hydroxyprogesterone, 880–881
  19-nortestosterone, 875, 880
Progestogens, 846, 907–908, **915–934**
Psychology, and menopause, 892
Pyridinoline, 822–823, 832

Quality of life, 949, 952–953
Quantitative computed tomography, 810–811

Radiogrammetry, 808

Salmon calcitonin, *see* Calcitonin
Secondary osteoporosis, 795
Serum enzymes, 818–820, 822
Serum lipids, **867–887**
  see also Lipoproteins
Serum markers—
  acid phosphatase, 821–822
  alkaline phosphatase, 818–819
  γ-carboxyglutamic acid, 822
  osteocalcin, 819
Sex steroid alternatives, and osteoporosis, **857–865**
Single photon absorptiometry, 808–809
Skeletal fragility, 785–788
  see also Fractures
Sodium fluoride, 862
Stanozolol, 863
Stress, 916–917
Subcutaneous oestrogens, 875

Tartrate-resistant acid phosphatase, 821–822
Tiludronates, 860–861
Transdermal oestrogen, 873–874
TRAP, *see* Plasma tartrate-resistant acid phosphatase
Trauma, risk for, 788–790

Urinary markers, 820–823
Urogenital atrophy, 891–892

Vaginal oestrogens, 872–873, 890
Vertebral fracture, 788–790
Vertebral osteoporosis, 825–826
Vitamin D metabolites, 861–862
VLDL, *see* Lipoproteins

X-ray absorptiometry, 810